Anne L. Strozier
Joyce Carpenter
Editors

Introduction
to Alternative
and Complementary
Therapies

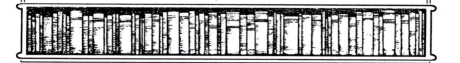

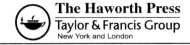

The Haworth Press
Taylor & Francis Group
New York and London

Introduction to Alternative and Complementary Therapies

HAWORTH Practical Practice in Mental Health
Terry S. Trepper
Senior Editor

Introduction
to Alternative
and Complementary
Therapies

Anne L. Strozier
Joyce Carpenter
Editors

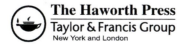

The Haworth Press
Taylor & Francis Group
New York and London

For more information on this book or to order, visit
http://www.haworthpress.com/store/product.asp?sku=5987

or call 1-800-HAWORTH (800-429-6784) in the United States and Canada
or (607) 722-5857 outside the United States and Canada
or contact orders@HaworthPress.com

The Haworth Press, Taylor & Francis Group, 270 Madison Avenue, New York, NY, 10016.

PUBLISHER'S NOTE
The development, preparation, and publication of this work has been undertaken with great care. However, the Publisher, employees, editors, and agents of The Haworth Press are not responsible for any errors contained herein or for consequences that may ensue from use of materials or information contained in this work. The Haworth Press is committed to the dissemination of ideas and information according to the highest standards of intellectual freedom and the free exchange of ideas. Statements made and opinions expressed in this publication do not necessarily reflect the views of the Publisher, Directors, management, or staff of The Haworth Press, or an endorsement by them.

Library of Congress Cataloging-in-Publication Data

Strozier, Anne L.
  Introduction to alternative and complementary therapies / Anne L. Strozier, Joyce Carpenter, editors.
      p. ; cm.
  Includes index.
  ISBN: 978-0-7890-2205-9 (hard : alk. paper)
  ISBN: 978-0-7890-2206-6 (soft : alk. paper)
  1. Alternative medicine. I. Strozier, Anne L. II. Carpenter, Joyce.
  [DNLM: 1. Complementary Therapies—methods. WB 890 I618 2007]

R733.I592 2007
615.5—dc22

                                                                              2007011206

CONTENTS

ABOUT THE EDITORS

Anne L. Strozier, PhD, MSW, is an Associate Professor in the School of Social Work at the University of South Florida. Dr. Strozier is also the Director of the Florida Kinship Center and a Licensed Psychologist in the state of Florida. She has used complementary and alternative approaches in her therapy practice for many years, has conducted research on the use of touch in psychotherapy, and has taught graduate social work classes and led professional workshops about complementary and alternative therapies.

Joyce Carpenter, MSW, grew up in Wallsend, an industrial town, in the North East of England. During her work as an elementary school teacher working with children in both urban and rural-based deprived neighborhoods, she recognized that many students failed to learn when taught by traditional methods. She began to use a multidisciplinary approach (incorporating poetry, music, drama, dance, art, and literature) to engage her students in their work. In 1992, she joined the faculty of the School of Social Work at the University of South Florida where she now works as an advisor and recruiter.

Introduction to Alternative and Complementary Therapies
© 2008 by The Haworth Press, Taylor & Francis Group. All rights reserved.
doi:10.1300/5987_a

CONTRIBUTORS

Pamela F. Beiler, MSW, LCSW, received her bachelor of science degree in communications from Bradley University, and her master of social work degree from the University of South Florida. She is currently a family therapist with The Horizons Program at The University of North Carolina School of Medicine at Chapel Hill. She has practiced and conducted research in areas including animal-assisted therapy, community mental health, domestic violence, kinship care, sexual abuse, and substance abuse.

Jeff Brantley, MD, is the founder and director of the mindfulness-based stress-reduction program in the Duke Center for Integrative Medicine. Dr. Brantley was born in North Carolina, attended Davidson College and the University of North Carolina at Chapel Hill School of Medicine. He trained in psychiatry at the University of California at Irvine, where he was first introduced to mindfulness meditation by Roger Walsh, MD, PhD. Dr. Brantley worked in both community psychiatry and private practice for 15 years, before accepting an invitation to develop a mindfulness-based stress reduction program as one of the initial offerings in the Integrative Medicine program that began at Duke Medical Center in 1998. Dr. Brantley is the author of *Calming Your Anxious Mind: How Mindfulness and Compassion Can Free You from Anxiety, Fear, and Panic,* and the co-author of *Five Good Minutes: 100 Morning Practices to Help You Stay Calm and Focused All Day Long.*

Laura A. Cherry, PhD, ATR-BC, received her BFA from Moore College of Art and Design and received her MA and PhD from Florida State University. She is an associate professor in the art department at Elizabeth City State University, part of the University of North Carolina system. Dr. Cherry has created and implemented

Introduction to Alternative and Complementary Therapies
© 2008 by The Haworth Press, Taylor & Francis Group. All rights reserved.
doi:10.1300/5987_b

xi

a number of art therapy programs for children with special needs in the Caribbean.

Irma Dosamantes-Beaudry, PhD, is a professor in the World Arts and Cultures Department of UCLA. Trained as a dance/movement therapist, clinical psychologist, and psychoanalyst, she directed the UCLA Graduate Dance/Movement Therapy Program at UCLA during 1977- 1999. She was elected President of the American Dance Therapy Association in 1980-1982 and the American Association for the Study of Mental Imagery during 1983-1984. In 1996 she was awarded a Lifetime Achievement Award for her contribution to the field of dance/movement therapy by the Chace Memorial Foundation. She served as the Editor-in-Chief of the *Arts in Psychotherapy Journal* during 1998-2003.

Dawn Doucette, MA, is a certified ayurvedic practitioner, has an MA in psychology from Columbia University, and is enrolled in the MSW program at the University of South Florida. Ms. Doucette has worked as a corporate executive, owned her own health care company, and served as an ayruvedic practitioner. She has lived and worked in many countries including India, Egypt, Guatemala, Thailand, Peru, Bolivia, and Costa Rica.

Trudy K. Duffy, PhD, is a certified practitioner and trainer in psychodrama, sociometry, and group psychotherapy. She uses active, expressive learning methods in teaching and in practice. She has worked with diverse populations in areas of prevention, health, developmental disabilities, and substance abuse. Her writings include the following: *Social Workers' Exercise of Authority in Court-Mandated Groups, White Gloves and Cracked Vases: How Metaphors Help Group Workers Construct New Perceptions and Responses, The Check-In and Other Go-Rounds in Groups,* and *Psychodrama in Early Recovery.* She is currently the co-chair of the clinical practice sequence and chair of the group work section at Boston University. She most recently completed a qualitative study of authority in groups from the perspective of the leaders—their experiences, beliefs, and frames for negotiating relationships with group members. The study elaborates methods for working with diverse involuntary client groups; it also illustrates the vulnerability that social workers in roles of high authority experience.

Aubrey H. Fine, EdD, faculty coordinator of Cal Poly Pomona's Center for Leadership and Service Learning and longtime professor in the College of Education and Integrative Studies. Born in Montreal, Canada, Fine received his undergraduate degree in psychology from Concordia University (Montreal) in 1977. He later obtained a master's in therapeutic recreation from the University of South Alabama (1978) and a doctorate in school psychology from the University of Cincinnati (1982). Fine has authored or co-authored eight books since 1988 and is working on a ninth. He has traveled throughout the United States and the world for over 70 conference presentations and scores of addresses and presentations. As both teacher and scholar, Fine is considered an expert in teaching, special education, child psychology, sport psychology, therapy, and gerontology.

Jennifer Jones, MM, MT-BC, has been a board-certified music therapist for over 12 years and has conducted music therapy with children, adolescents, and adults in Tennessee, Florida, and Pennsylvania in acute and extended care psychiatric and substance abuse service agencies. Her recent national and international music therapy conference presentations have included sessions and research on songwriting methods, aspects of music therapist's nonverbal communication, and practical research design for clinicians. She served on the board of directors for the Southeastern Region of the American Music Therapy Association for four years. After serving on the faculty at Tennessee Tech University, she expects to finish her doctorate in music therapy at Florida State University in 2006.

Erin Kuhn, MSW, has graduated from Florida State University with a bachelor's degree in psychology and the University of South Florida with a master's degree in social work. She has worked with children in the school system and adults in substance abuse.

Ann Lindell, CPA, developed interest in religious philosophies in the 1970s while studying at the University of South Florida. She furthered her education in Eastern religions through classes at Naropa University, numerous workshops and retreats while raising her children, working as a community volunteer and activist and practicing as a CPA. Her mindfulness meditation practice has been reinforced through her involvement in a Buddhist Sangha which studies the teachings of *Thich Nhat Hanh*. She currently lives with her husband

and children in Tampa and is working on her master's in social work at the University of South Florida.

Perie J. Longo, PhD, is the current president of the National Association for Poetry Therapy (NAPT), a registered poetry therapist and a mentor/supervisor for those seeking credentials in the field, and a marriage and family therapist (MFT) in private practice. She directs poetry therapy at Sanctuary Psychiatric Centers in Santa Barbara, CA, as well as Hospice of Santa Barbara. She has published articles in *The Journal of Poetry Therapy,* and is the author of two collections of poetry, *Milking the Earth* and *The Privacy of Wind.*

Catherine E. Randall, MSW, LMT, has been a licensed massage therapist since 2001, and received her master's degree in social work from the University of South Florida in 2006. She has used touch therapies with adults diagnosed with physical and emotional disorders. She has worked with children in a medical environment, and has experience using craniosacral therapy with children.

Mary P. Van Hook, PhD, is a professor and the director of a school of social work. She received her MSW from Columbia University and her PhD from Rutgers University. In addition to teaching social work at several univerities, she has also worked extensively in the areas of mental health and family services. Her interest in the value of addressing spirituality as part of holistic social work practice grew out of her experience of working with individuals from a variety of cultural and religious backgrounds. She has presented workshops and published in the area of spirituality as a resource for social workers. She co-edited the book *Spirituality Within Religious Traditions in Social Work Practice.*

Chapter 1

Introduction

Anne L. Strozier

Psychotherapists rely on a variety of therapeutic approaches including psychodynamic, analytic, humanistic, systems, cognitive, narrative, and solution-focused treatment. These therapies use different techniques to help clients, ranging from reflection to interpretation, education to confrontation, and mirroring to seeking solutions. Though these techniques vary a great deal, they have one thing in common: they are verbal interventions.

This book presents therapeutic interventions that are complementary or alternative to therapists' verbal work with clients, adding depth, breadth, and creativity to therapeutic practice. These approaches rely less on verbal interventions and more on methods that utilize the client's mind in relationship with other senses such as touch, sound, movement, and visual stimuli. Complementary and alternative approaches transcend traditional models and integrate the body and mind through a holistic therapeutic process.

WHY SHOULD I READ THIS BOOK?

Why would you want to read this book about alternative and complementary therapeutic approaches? One reason is to provide new options for you when one of your clients gets "stuck" in treatment. Complementary and alternative approaches can open up new avenues for working with clients at a roadblock. For example, imagine that

Introduction to Alternative and Complementary Therapies
© 2008 by The Haworth Press, Taylor & Francis Group. All rights reserved.
doi:10.1300/5987_01

your client has made progress during psychodynamic therapy, but now is reerecting defenses such as intellectualization. What can you do? You can try your usual techniques and approaches, but what if they fail? A complete change in therapeutic approaches, even for a short while, may allow your client to resolve the resistance and move forward in therapy. You may decide to use art therapy, music therapy, or mindfulness techniques. This book will explain the basics of how therapies such as these work and will provide examples for utilizing them in treatment.

Complementary approaches can also be used in conjunction with traditional therapies during the entire counseling experience. For example, if you are a cognitive therapist, you might decide to introduce poetry therapy to a client as an adjunct to therapy. Such a complementary technique can provide rich and valuable material for the therapist and for the client on the road to self-discovery and healing.

Another reason to learn about these complementary and alternative approaches is that according to recent research the most effective psychotherapeutic treatments are those that are tailored to meet the specific needs of individual clients. This means that a therapist, rather than fitting the client to match a given therapeutic approach, should select from a repertoire of therapeutic approaches to find those that will best fit *that client*. Reading this book will allow you to select from a greater breadth and depth of therapeutic approaches. With this increased knowledge of treatment modalities, the likelihood of finding the appropriate treatment for each client will be greatly enhanced.

Alternative and complementary modalities of treatment also challenge our thinking. These new approaches conceptualize client problems and the treatment process differently. Most of us counsel clients using well-established and well-practiced frameworks. Learning about complementary and alternative therapies opens up our thinking to be able to see new schema for both understanding and treating our clients. Thinking in these new ways helps us to continue to grow as professionals while providing our clients with innovative ways to achieve their personal goals.

Last, complementary therapies can be fun! Clients often enjoy the opportunity to grow in a new way, and likewise, we feel alive and vital when we grow professionally. Therapy is more enjoyable and probably a more successful endeavor when not only our clients but also we, as therapists, are challenged and growing.

WHAT ARE ALTERNATIVE
AND COMPLEMENTARY METHODS?

The approaches in this book are based largely on complementary and alternative medicine, commonly referred to as CAM. CAM is a group of nontraditional medical systems, treatments, and products that are used to either accompany or replace conventional medical treatments. Complementary approaches to psychotherapy are considered part of this larger system.

CAM contains five subcategories, called domains, which help further define the objective and intent of these treatments. The five domains are: *alternative medical systems, mind-body interventions, biologically based therapies, manipulative and body-based methods,* and *energy therapies.*

Alternative medical systems are considered complete medical sciences with their origin in ancient eastern cultures such as traditional Chinese medicine and India's medical science, ayurveda. *Mind-body interventions* are those therapies that help patients facilitate their own healing process through meditation, prayer, and the creative arts. *Biologically based therapies* are products such as dietary supplements and herbal products which contain substances found in nature that are believed to work in collaboration with the body's own biochemical makeup. *Manipulative body-based interventions* are physical treatments such as massage and chiropractic manipulation that move specific body parts to facilitate a healing reaction. *Energy therapies,* such as Reiki and Therapeutic Touch, work to balance the energy fields that exist both inside and around the body, typically without using physical touch.

DOES ANYONE REALLY USE ALTERNATIVE/
COMPLEMENTARY THERAPIES?

Yes! In fact, alternative and complementary therapies are gaining popularity every year as people learn about them and the evidence of their effectiveness in treating different conditions increases. Because of the popularity and success of these therapies, the U.S. government established the National Center for Complementary and Alternative Medicine (NCCAM). NCCAM and the National Center for Health Statistics have tracked patients' personal experiences with CAM therapies to understand actual usage. Between 1990 and 1997, visits to CAM practitioners increased almost 50 percent. A 2002 study found that 62 percent of adult Americans reported using at least one type of CAM therapy in the last 12 months. A 1997 consumer report found that at least $36 billion was spent by the U.S. government on CAM therapies in 1997, and at least $12 billion was spent by individuals with no insurance coverage. In 1994, legislation categorizing herbal medicines as food supplements opened the distribution markets and it has been estimated that sales of herbal products have doubled since then.

With this increased interest and availability, CAM therapies are used by diverse populations for a range of illnesses. Studies show that CAM is most often used by women, hospitalized individuals, and former smokers. CAM use is not mediated by race: studies found consistent use in Asian, black, Hispanic, and white populations. The most widely used domains, making up 95 percent of usage, are *mind-body medicine* (including meditation, prayer, and cognitive therapies), *biologically based* practices (including dietary supplements and herbal products), and *body-based therapies* (including massage and chiropractic manipulation). The five most common health conditions treated with CAM are back pain, head cold, neck pain, joint pain, and depression.

Medical centers and universities have joined efforts to integrate CAM therapies into conventional medical facilities. This integration not only helps make CAM accessible to the public but also provides a venue for research and education. Seventy-three medical schools now offer classes in CAM and the recently formed Consortium of Academic Health Centers for Integrative Medicine reports that 27 of the top medical centers in the United States are collaborating on research, clinical care, and education for the advancement of CAM. *MedBioWorld* lists over 50 associations and organizations and over 60 professional journals dedicated to the education and practice of CAM treatments.

A great deal of research is currently underway to evaluate the effectiveness of complementary and alternative approaches. You will read about some of that research in this book.

OVERVIEW OF THE BOOK

This book will introduce you to a number of the most noteworthy complementary and alternative treatment approaches researched, developed, and implemented in recent years. The CAM approaches selected are ones that are particularly relevant to psychotherapists. Each chapter is written by a leading expert in that field and includes a description of the approach, research evidence about its effectiveness, guidelines on how to use the therapy in practice, and case examples.

We begin the book with the chapter "Mindfulness, Meditation, and Health." The chapter includes a discussion of the mind-body relationship, citing research that demonstrates the strong influence of our mind on emotional and physical well-being. Dr. Jeff Brantley, Dawn Doucette, and Ann Lindell have written a clear and thoughtful chapter describing the research efforts in the areas of mindfulness, meditation, and methods for living a focused and aware life.

Dr. Mary Van Hook's chapter on spirituality teaches the reader about the collaborative healing relationship between counseling and spirituality. Meanings of words such as spirituality, religion, and healing are addressed. In addition, Dr. Van Hook responds to the question of why spirituality and religion should be included in the counseling process and explores numerous ways to incorporate spirituality within counseling. Her chapter's examples of using spirituality as a complementary intervention demonstrate the benefits that the counselor and client gain from using counseling models which stress the meaning of spirituality in the lives of clients.

Dr. Perie Longo's compelling chapter on poetry as therapy includes her experience with poetry's role for clients in group therapy as well as individual treatment. Many of her clients' poems are included, which makes the chapter not only fascinating to read, but also clarifies poetry's role as a therapeutic approach. Dr. Longo explores the healing components of poetry such as rhythm, metaphor, repetition, words chosen, form, and shape, which join together in helping the therapist frame questions to process the client's meaning. Longo explains how clients find a voice through their own poetry.

The next chapter, which is on art therapy, is written by Dr. Laura Cherry. Dr. Cherry reassures the reader that talent in art is not a necessary component for using art therapy. Cherry not only describes research studies on art therapy but also presents very practical information such as the art materials required for art therapy. Cherry ends the chapter with a moving and elucidating case example of art therapy with a six-year-old boy with cerebral palsy.

Psychodrama, as explained by Dr. Trudy Duffy, is a therapy wherein participants act out issues from their own lives to relieve mental problems or emotional conflicts, and to strengthen interpersonal relationships. Dr. Duffy explains how the use of spontaneity and creativity encourage participants to express themselves while finding innovative ways to approach the issues in their lives. Different techniques that can be used in psychodrama, including role reversal, doubling, mirroring, soliloquy, concretizing, empty chair, future projection, and dream presentation are described. Dr. Duffy cites several case examples of psychodrama to demonstrate its versatility for use in different groups and settings.

Dr. Dosamantes-Beaudry discusses how dance/movement therapy (DMT) heals by allowing participants to work with unknown forces both within themselves and in the environment, offering a means for participants to vent negative emotions while providing a safe environment to act out these behaviors, giving an outlet to voice changes in role or status, and finally allowing clients to be an integral part of their cultural group. This chapter investigates DMT as a style of psychotherapy that uses the body as a means of expressing conflicts and desires, while promoting self development.

In the chapter that follows the one by Dr. Dosamantes-Beaudry, Jennifer Jones establishes the concept of music as a language of emotions, a therapy that gives expression to inarticulate thoughts and feelings. Jones discusses how music therapy's unique qualities of being a social, sensory, and organized meaningful experience promote positive changes in the client with limited verbal processes.

The chapter on animal-assisted therapy, written by Dr. Aubrey Fine and Pamela Beiler, presents research regarding the healing aspects of animals in therapy, including physical and psychosocial benefits. Fine and Beiler address basic foundation strategies to consider when incorporating animal-assisted therapy in psychotherapy: animals as a social lubricant, animals as a catalyst for emotion, animals as adjuncts to clinicians, and animals as part of the therapeutic environment. Case examples of client-animal interactions as well as Fine's research findings create a greater understanding of the benefits of animals assisting therapy.

The last chapter presents an overview of various uses of touch in therapy: touch during the psychotherapeutic process, Reiki, therapeutic touch, and even massage therapy. Dr. Anne Strozier, Catherine Randall, and Erin Kuhn describe each of these therapeutic interventions and the research studies evaluating their effectiveness. A discussion of important legal and ethical implications and considerations is included. Case examples bring touch therapies to life.

The book presents an array of resources for you: Web sites, state and national organizations, accrediting boards, and more. We hope these will provide you with enough information to further research any complementary or alternative approach that especially appeals to you. This book is intended to pique your interest, light your curiosity, and perhaps inspire you to learn more about one or two of these approaches in depth. For, while we hope that you will enjoy learning about the complementary and alternative therapies and gain much insight into them through this book, it is essential to know that this book is not intended as an in-depth training manual for the therapies presented. If you plan to incorporate a complementary or alternative approach into your current or future practice, you will need to pursue further education and training in that area. We hope you feel intrigued, excited, and challenged when reading this book, inspired to learn more about these very important complementary and alternative approaches to psychotherapy.

Chapter 2

Mindfulness, Meditation, and Health

Jeff Brantley
Dawn Doucette
Ann Lindell

INTRODUCTION

Human beings have an innate potential to realize deep awareness of their thoughts, actions, and interactions. When this awareness is experienced in each moment in a nonjudgmental way, one is said to have become mindful. *Mindfulness* is a consciousness that is achieved by paying attention and being present in one's life.

For literally thousands of years, individuals in many cultures have cultivated mindfulness explicitly through the activity of meditation. Motivations for meditation practice are usually linked to the goals of healing and transformation. The practice of mindfulness meditation emphasizes nonjudgmental acceptance and interested awareness. Ancient methods of meditation aimed at developing mindfulness have evolved in Western medicine and psychology for the purposes of health and healing. Through the years, meditation practices have evolved from their original cultural and religious contexts and become available to anyone seeking enhancement to medical treatment.

In this chapter, the history of mindfulness, the role of meditation in achieving mindfulness, and the effects of mindfulness on health and healing will be discussed. Illustrative case studies and practical exercises are also included in this chapter.

Introduction to Alternative and Complementary Therapies
© 2008 by The Haworth Press, Taylor & Francis Group. All rights reserved.
doi:10.1300/5987_02

UNDERSTANDING THE CONCEPT
OF MINDFULNESS

Mindfulness is an activity that directs attention and cultivates awareness in particular ways for particular purposes (Goleman, 1977; Feldman, 1998). Jon Kabat-Zinn (2003), founder of the mindfulness-based stress reduction program and a prolific writer on mindfulness, provides an operational working definition of mindfulness as "the awareness that emerges through paying attention on purpose, in the present moment, and nonjudgmentally, to the unfolding experience moment by moment" (Kabat-Zinn, 2003, p. 144).

The meaning of mindfulness can be clarified by breaking down the definition of mindfulness and focusing on its key words: awareness, purpose, nonjudgmental, and present moment. Mindfulness is an "awareness" that occurs when all the distractions of life are removed and one is able to fully focus on the here and now. Mindfulness is driven by "purpose" or intent to create that feeling of awareness. Mindfulness requires a "nonjudgmental" perspective similar to observation, in which one watches and does not engage. Mindfulness occurs in the "present moment," avoiding the disturbances of the wandering mind.

Mindfulness is often associated with Buddhist teachings and is believed to be a fundamental principle across all Buddhist traditions. However, mindfulness is actually a universal concept that transcends religious teachings or any particular philosophy. Buddhism has helped create traditions or practices to cultivate mindfulness, and in that regard it is a Buddhist teaching, but the inherent capacity of all humans to create mindfulness makes it universally accessible.

Mindful attention can be applied to any aspect of experience including thoughts, actions, and interactions. Mindfulness heightens the experience of inner life events of emotions, thoughts, and sensations. One can also bring mindful attention to the outer life, including relationships and social experiences. This increase in presence makes both the joys and difficulties in one's life more visible, and hence, easier to navigate. The clarity obtained through mindfulness increases one's wisdom to help make life choices. Even without calling it "mindfulness," most people have had experiences of being present, and can appreciate the power of connection and the feeling of being alive that such presence brings.

CULTIVATING MINDFULNESS
THROUGH MEDITATION

Mindfulness requires training the mind to let go of thoughts by creating a peaceful awareness that allows insight to follow. To that end, mindfulness is often cultivated through the practice of meditation.

Meditation is one of the most ancient of human activities, and has been one of the most widely practiced of the *mind-body therapies* currently available to Western health care practitioners (National Institute of Health, 2004). Meditation is a training of the mind that frees the mind from clutter and creates a peaceful space that allows one to develop awareness.

There are thousands of methods and techniques for practicing meditation which exist within larger traditions of meditation embedded in specific cultural, spiritual, and historical contexts. Yet despite these apparent differences, meditation traditions share certain core principles. Meditation teacher Christina Feldman (1998) notes that all meditative traditions share four common principles: *attention, awareness, understanding,* and *compassion.*

Attention provides for the cultivation of intention and sets the stage for one to begin the meditation with an open and clear mind. Awareness grounds meditation in the present moment and allows for one to participate in a knowing and nonjudgmental way. Understanding brings inner wisdom to the meditation and compassion allows the individual to look beyond the self and expand the meditation to include the collective nature of all beings. Based on these four principles, practicing meditation means to take a period of time for practice and make a determined effort. During that time it is essential to establish attention in the present moment, relax into a consciousness that is open, maintain attitudes of kindness and compassion, and acknowledge an understanding of inner wisdom.

Meditation Practices

According to many authorities, meditation practices can be divided into two categories: *concentrative* or *awareness* practices (Boorstein, 1996). In fact, all meditation practices utilize elements of both concentration and awareness, but it is the relative emphasis that a particular method places on a technique that distinguishes one from another.

Whatever the practice emphasis, on a deeper level of human life the aim of meditation has to do with transformation and healing.

Concentration meditation provides two outcomes: concentration and relaxation. During concentrative meditation one typically focuses on a single object: a mantra, a word or phrase to be repeated, a sensation (such as the breath), or a physical object. The mind often wanders from the object of attention, and one must calmly return attention to the chosen object. It often takes thousands of times before the mind becomes focused on that object. When the mind wanders, it is not a mistake but a habit of the mind which needs to be redirected. When the mind wanders to a thought, one merely disregards the thought and focuses back on the object. Meditation is a technique that trains the mind to be stable. The best way to train one's attention to be stable and steady is to practice focusing attention and repeatedly returning it to the object with an attitude of patience and kindness. This is the beginning practice of meditation.

Concentration meditation brings a feeling of peace and calm in mind and body. Harvard cardiologist, Herbert Benson (1993), while studying practitioners of transcendental meditation, coined the phrase "the relaxation response" to describe the calmness and tranquility in mind and body elicited by the practice of meditation.

Meditation teachers for thousands of years have acknowledged the importance of calmness and ease in the practice of meditation. Relaxation meditation, with its roots in Hinduism, is often described using the word *shamatha,* which is Sanskrit for "dwelling in tranquility" (Schuhmacher & Woerner, 1994, p. 314). Buddhist texts also note the benefits of meditation practices that emphasize concentrated attention. Meditation teacher and psychotherapist Sylvia Boorstein notes that the practice of single focus attention in meditation produces a sense of ease, balance, and relaxation. This is a state traditional Buddhist texts call "malleability of mind" (Boorstein, 1996, p. 58).

Awareness meditation includes those methods that emphasize present moment awareness or mindfulness and is often referred to as mindfulness meditation. Mindfulness meditation is the foundation for developing mindfulness and is most often used in mental health settings when utilizing mindfulness in programs and interventions. Mindfulness meditation differs from concentration meditation by observing the changing thoughts occurring from inner and outer stimuli (Baer, 2003).

While mindfulness has been developed by human beings throughout history, and in many cultures, Buddhists have added significantly to the technology of meditation practices that emphasize mindfulness. Mindfulness meditation is central to, and can be found throughout the *Vipassana,* Tibetan, and Zen traditions of Buddhism. However, the secular use of mindfulness often eliminates the central theme in Buddhist mindfulness meditation practice which is to generate compassion for all beings. Jon Kabat-Zinn (2003) argues that the acceptance of Buddhist tradition is irrelevant to mindfulness practice since mindfulness is truly a universal concept. The Western approach to mindfulness meditation focuses more on training the mind to connect with present experience.

One example of mindfulness meditation exists in the *Vipassana* tradition. In *Vipassana,* mindfulness meditation is also known as insight meditation. Meditation instructions in this tradition often emphasize cultivation of mindfulness through careful attention to minute details of experience, always with a nonjudgmental and accepting attitude. It is common for a *Vipassana* retreat to last 7 to 10 days during which time one practices meditation in total silence for the duration of the retreat. This practice allows time to train the mind and cultivate a heightened sense of awareness and insight. A popular teacher in this tradition is S. N. Goenka (2005), who explains *Vipassana* practice thus:

> Vipassana is a way of self transformation through self-observation. It focuses on the deep interconnection between mind and body, which can be experienced directly by disciplined attention to the physical sensations that form the life of the body, and that continuously interconnect and condition the life of the mind. It is this observation-based, self-exploratory journey to the common root of mind and body that dissolves mental impurity, resulting in a balanced mind full of love and compassion. (p. 1)

Though awareness meditation moves beyond relaxation and into exploration, it depends on the technique of concentration to calm and focus the mind. During insight meditation, one explores sensations in the body, thoughts, or feelings, and begins to observe the nature and origin of such sensations. Through this awareness, a heightened sense of self-understanding and acceptance is achieved. Meditation is recommended for the teacher as well as the student, for the healthy as well as the unhealthy, and for the spiritual as well as the secular.

THE HISTORY OF MINDFULNESS AND MEDITATION

Through out the first part of this chapter the connection between mindfulness and meditation has been explored by discussing the intent of mindfulness and the use of meditation to help achieve it. Because the relationship between mindfulness and meditation is so interconnected, it is almost impossible to separate the two. Mindfulness and meditation in their historical context have the same relationship: they are interdependently woven together.

The majority of meditation practices that are taught in current therapeutic contexts have their origins in traditional Eastern philosophies. Buddha taught mindfulness to his followers, as detailed in two core discourses: the *Anapanasati* Sutra (Rosenberg, 1998) and the *Satipatthana* Sutra (Smith, 1999). These two texts are the foundation of Buddhist teaching on mindfulness and describe how unexamined behaviors and an untrained mind can contribute to human suffering. They also explain how meditation practices aimed at calming the mind, providing clarity, and opening the heart allow for healing and transformation (Kabat-Zinn, 2003). For over 2,500 years, mindfulness has been at the center of Buddhist meditation (Hanh, 1999; Gunaratana, 1992).

Eastern religion, and particularly Buddhism, flourished in the United States during the last half of the twentieth century, and with it, an interest in meditation. The Communist invasion of Asia and the subsequent exile of His Holiness the Dalai Lama from Tibet created an open road to bring the teachings out of the East and into the West (Murphy & Donovan, 1997). The Beatles' association with the Indian Hindu Maharishi Mahesh Yogi in the 1960s and the interest in consciousness due to the psychedelic revolution led the way to an interest in another Eastern practice, transcendental meditation.

American Interest in Meditation

In the 1950s, a major leap occurred in American interest in both meditation and Asian philosophy (Taylor, 1997). Frederic Speigelberg, a Stanford religion professor, opened the California Institute of Asian Studies in 1951. Alan Watts, a Zen student, joined the faculty and began exploring the interface of Asian and Western culture in his writing and teachings. And, notably, in the 1950s, the Zen teacher D. T. Suzuki came to America from Japan. His seminars had a wide influence on cultural leaders such as Thomas Merton, psychoanalyst Karen Horney, and the popular writer J. D. Salinger. His teachings became widely translated and available to American audiences.

In the 1960s, cultural impact from the Vietnam War, the explosion of interest in psychedelics and mind-expanding drugs, and the development of an American counterculture combined and led to widespread interest and experimentation in all forms of meditation. This expansion also resulted in increased attention on the role of meditation and mindfulness and its relationship to physical and psychological well-being. One of the first pundits to address this connection, Alan Watts (1961), stated:

> The main resemblance between these Eastern ways of life and Western psychotherapy is in the concern of both with bringing about changes of consciousness, changes in our ways of feeling our own existence, and our relation to human society and the natural world. The psychotherapist has, for the most part, been interested in changing the consciousness of peculiarly disturbed individuals. The disciplines of Buddhism and Taoism are, however, concerned with changing the consciousness of normal, socially adjusted people. (p. 3)

Alan Watts was prescient in his recognition of the role of Eastern philosophy in Western medicine and psychology for the purposes of healing. Unlike traditional Western medicine, which focuses on diseases of the sick, the holistic nature of Eastern medicine is also relevant for the diseases of normal life of the well individual. Meditation in its development of mindfulness is a useful practice to ease the ubiquitous suffering of our human existence. Western psychologists and therapists have become increasingly interested in how individuals practicing meditation might evoke changes in consciousness that have clinical benefits.

MINDFULNESS AND HEALTH

Mindfulness meditation is cultivated from a base of relaxed attention from which deeper awareness of the contents of experience emerges. As this attention and deeper awareness strengthen, a base for cognitive learning and understanding develops. Through instruction and practice, meditation teaches one to recognize the repetitive patterns of thinking, emotions, and bodily reactions, and inquire into them. Over time, recognition, understanding, and the resulting reduced reactivity can lead to more adaptive and skillful responses to stress or other demands of an illness.

According to Hayes, Strosahl, and Wilson (1999), psychological therapies with mindfulness or insight meditation techniques at their core have evolved out of earlier behavioral and cognitive models. These newer therapies differ in that they often focus on techniques not traditionally used such as "mindfulness, acceptance, the therapeutic relationship, values, spirituality, meditation focusing on the present moment, emotional deepening, and similar topics" (Hayes et al., 1999, p. xiii).

When mindfulness is practiced in the context of health and healing, a person begins to develop a different relationship to his or her experience around wellness and disease. This includes relationships to both the inner subjective experience and the outer social experience. Mindfulness can increase the awareness of how emotions affect the body as well as connect one to the consequences of lifestyle on health. As mindfulness training has been offered to people with a wide variety of health issues, a robust public and professional interest in mindfulness has developed.

Mindfulness has been reported to have a positive effect on physiological symptoms such as blood pressure, pain, and immune functioning. This approach can induce a feeling of relaxation, increasing one's ability to deal with life's stressors simply by being aware. It is this awareness that can change the way in which both body and mind respond, allowing the body the freedom to self-heal. As well, an increase in mindfulness can bring a heightened awareness to the effect of lifestyle choice on both the physical and emotional body, cultivating the ability to make healthier choices.

Since the 1960s, Western clinicians familiar with mindfulness from personal experience with Buddhist meditation have been exploring effective applications of mindfulness in different clinical settings. Examples include research in the use of *Vipassana* meditation in substance abuse treatment (Marlatt, 2002), and applications of acceptance and nonjudging awareness in a variety of psychotherapeutic settings (Hayes et al., 1999; Epstein, 1996; Brach, 2003).

As Marlatt (1994) points out, a variety of potential applications exist for mindfulness training. These include exposure and desensitization, thought monitoring, relaxation, and acceptance. There is also increasing evidence that meditation may influence physiological reactivity.

CLINICAL APPLICATIONS OF MINDFULNESS

Mindfulness can be used in collaboration with traditional psychology models as well as with Western medical protocols. Therapists have explored the use of mindfulness meditation in stress reduction, medical conditions commonly associated with stress such as hypertension, and mindfulness as a means for managing symptoms of personality disorders. The following is a description of three techniques that apply mindfulness to health and well-being: mindfulness-based stress reduction, dialectical behavior therapy, and mindfulness-based cognitive therapy.

Mindfulness-Based Stress Reduction (MBSR)

In 1979, Jon Kabat-Zinn and his colleagues at the University of Massachusetts Medical Center in Worcester, began offering a program in mindfulness training to patients referred to their clinic. They sought to make mindfulness available through meditation practice in a nonsectarian way focused on stress reduction and health enhancement rather than on any particular spiritual or religious form.

The program had a twofold aim (Kabat-Zinn, 2003). First, MBSR was a vehicle through which medical patients could begin to assume a greater degree of responsibility for their own health and well-being through the practice of mindfulness. Second, the approach was meant to be one that, if successful, could be adapted to a wide variety of settings in clinics and hospitals.

The MBSR model is intended as a complement—not a substitute—for any treatment an individual is receiving. In this model, participants with a wide variety of medical and stress-related conditions attend a weekly class in which they are taught a number of practices aimed at developing and applying relaxation and mindfulness to their unique situation or condition. They are encouraged to practice formal meditation aimed at developing mindfulness of the inner life, body sensations, and ordinary activities of daily life such as walking, eating, and doing chores. In addition, they are taught simple poses from Hatha yoga, and they make a commitment to practice at home up to an hour daily. Through class discussion and presentations, participants learn about stress, its effects, and styles of coping as they begin to establish mindfulness in the ongoing situations of daily life. Throughout the class cycle, emphasis is placed upon precisely directing attention, and cultivating a less goal-directed, nonjudging observation of both inner and outer experience. Typically the class extends over a period of eight weeks, and includes a daylong intensive session (the Day of Mindfulness) near the end of the course.

Benefits from participation in MBSR program have been reported in the literature. Some examples focusing on anxiety and depression are listed here:

- Pre-medical and medical students were placed into two groups in a randomized waitlist format for training in MBSR. Students receiving training in mindfulness meditation reported significant reductions in anxiety and depression (Shapiro, Schwartz, & Bonner, 1998).
- Reibel and colleagues (Reibel, Greeson, Brainard, & Rosenzweig, 2001) reported significant reductions in anxiety and depression in a prospective, observational study of a group of medical patients representing a variety of diagnoses.
- In a randomized wait-list controlled study of a group of patients with various types of cancer, Speca and colleagues (Speca, Carlson, Goodey, & Angen, 2000) found significant reductions in anxiety and depression scares following training in the MBSR approach.

- Tacon and colleagues (Tacon, McComb, Caldera, & Randolph, 2003) reported reductions of anxiety in a small, randomized trial study of a group of women with heart disease.
- Significant reductions in anxiety and depression among individuals with generalized anxiety and panic disorder have been reported (Kabat-Zinn et al., 1992). These reductions were maintained at a three-year follow-up.

In addition to reduction of anxiety and depression, mindfulness approaches grounded in MBSR have been used with patients experiencing generalized anxiety disorder, panic disorder, panic disorder with agoraphobia (Kabat-Zinn, 1982); relapsing depression (Teasdale et al., 2000); eating disorders (Kristeller & Hallett, 1999); cancer (Speca et al., 2000); chronic pain (Kabat-Zinn et al., 1985, 1986); fibromyalgia (Kaplan et al., 1993; Goldenberg et al., 1994; Weissbecker et al., 2002); and psoriasis (Kabat-Zinn et al., 1998).

Dialectical Behavior Therapy (DBT)

Marsha Linehan developed dialectical behavior therapy (DBT) in the 1970s as an approach to the treatment of borderline personality disorder (BPD) and suicidal behavior that "all but demands mindfulness as a critical element" (Hayes, Follette, & Linehan, 2004, p. 31). Recognizing that clients with BPD were particularly sensitive to criticism and were highly emotional, a method was developed that would "hold both acceptance and change in the therapy simultaneously, a synthesis that, when found, could engender both new client change and new acceptance" (Hayes, Follette, & Linehan, 2004, p. 38). Linehan linked the skills of acceptance directly to a mindfulness perspective drawn from Zen Buddhism (Hayes, Follette, & Linehan, 2004; Linehan, 1993a,b).

According to this approach, dialectics has to do with "the process or art of reasoning by discussion of conflicting ideas" (*Merriam-Webster's Dictionary,* 1997, p. 216). DBT encourages the client through a process of self-acceptance while helping to change harmful behavior. DBT uses mindfulness practices to help the client learn acceptance, focus on the moment, and embrace reality without judgment. Radical acceptance is the term that describes this approach that is both an outcome and an activity (Hayes, Follette, & Linehan, 2004).

These mindfulness skills support an accurate and nonjudgmental observation of experience, including one's thoughts and emotions, while behavioral therapies then address changes that are needed. DBT uses skills training, cognitive modification, contingency management, and exposure-based therapies.

DBT has been clinically evaluated for the treatment of BPD, bulimia nervosa, substance abuse, depression, eating disorders, and self-injurious behavior. A controlled study done in the Netherlands of randomly selected participants with BPD found DBT had significantly superior results on treatment retention with high-risk behavior. This and other empirical studies have shown promising results but are considered preliminary at this time (Hayes et al., 2004).

Mindfulness-Based Cognitive Therapy (MBCT)

Segal, Williams, and Teasdale developed their MBCT model in response to the need for an effective method of preventing or reducing relapse in patients with major depressive disorder (MDD). They initially met in 1989 at the World Congress of Cognitive Therapy and discussed their interest in psychological research, treatment of depression, and cognitive therapy (Segal, Williams, & Teasdale, 2002, p. 4). The researchers discussed the high incidence of MDD with its high rate of relapse. Judd, Akiskal, and Paulus (1997) found that more than 80 percent of previously diagnosed patients with MDD experienced relapse with an average of four episodes. In 2002, Segal, Williams, and Teasdale published *Mindfulness-Based Cognitive Therapy for Depression: A New Approach to Preventing Relapse,* a book that describes the development of a mindfulness-based cognitive therapy (MBCT) specifically geared toward the treatment of depression.

A leading model of cognitive theory, as developed by Aaron T. Beck in the 1960s, is based on the idea that underlying dysfunctional attitudes and assumptions are the cause of depression (Segal, Williams, & Teasdale, 2002, p. 21). Cognitive therapy is meant to help patients recognize these negative thoughts and more accurately address them. Some of the techniques used to treat depression are thought monitoring, cognitive rehearsal, generating alternative options, and noticing and dealing with dysfunctional attitudes.

It had originally been assumed that the dysfunctional thinking associated with MDD was an enduring trait that would contribute to increased vulnerability for relapse. However, Beck's Dysfunctional Attitude Scale disproved this theory after a review of over 40 studies showed no difference between those subjects with no depressive disorder, and those with depression in a recovery or non-relapsed state (Ingram, Miranda, & Segal, 1998). Teasdale, in response to these findings, reflected on the following:

> Although the explicit emphasis in cognitive therapy is on changing thought content, we realized that it was equally possible that, when successful, this treatment led implicitly to changes in patients' relationships to their negative thoughts and feelings. Specifically, as a result of repeatedly identifying negative thoughts as they arose and standing back from them to evaluate the accuracy of their content, patients often made a more general shift in their perspective on negative thoughts and feelings. Rather than regarding thoughts as necessarily true or as an aspect of the self, patients switched to a perspective within which negative thoughts and feelings could be seen as passing events in the mind that were neither necessarily valid reflections of reality nor central aspects of the self. The importance of such "distancing or decentering" had previously been recognized in discussions of cognitive therapy, but usually as a means to an end, changing thought content, rather than an end in itself. (Segal, Williams, & Teasdale, 2002, p. 38)

Teasdale, Segal, and Williams were aware of the mindfulness training being used by Marsha Linehan (DBT) and Jon Kabat-Zinn (MBSR) discussed earlier in the chapter (Hayes, Follette, & Linehan, 2004, p. 51). Recognizing that mindfulness training works to change the *relationship* with thoughts, as compared to traditional cognitive therapy which works to change the *content* of the thoughts, they combined cognitive therapy approaches with the mindfulness training format of MBSR and called it mindfulness-based cognitive therapy (MBCT). In this approach, MBCT teaches clients to observe their thoughts and feelings in a nonjudgmental way, as mental events that come and go. By not identifying with distorted thoughts and feelings, the individual is believed to be better able to resist the escalation of ruminations and negative thoughts characteristic of relapsing depression (Teasdale et al., 1995). Subsequent research in MBCT supports this view, and results suggest significant benefits in this method for individuals with relapsing major depression (Teasdale et al., 2000). The MBCT approach is available as an eight-week group intervention based largely on the MBSR format with an emphasis on mindfulness practices (Segal, Williams, & Teasdale, 2002). The authors encourage a mindfulness meditation practice for their MBCT group leaders and adhere to one of the principal tenets of MBSR, that the instructor has a strongly developed and ongoing personal mindfulness or meditation practice (Segal, Williams, & Teasdale, 2002, p. 84).

CASE STUDIES

Bill's Story

Bill has symptoms of generalized anxiety disorder. He lives with intense worry and imagines a variety of terrible things happening in almost every situation he enters. Over the years of living with this condition, Bill has come to hate the worry and fears he imagines. Worse, he has come to be a harsh critic of himself, blaming himself for the continuing episodes of anxiety and its disturbances in his life.

After Bill began to practice mindfulness, he started to notice the patterns of his thoughts and the habits of criticizing and judgment that arose whenever the anxiety and worry came. He remembered to practice nonjudging as he learned to establish attention on his own thoughts and feelings. After a while, Bill began to see that his judgments were just another set of thoughts passing through the present moment, and could relax a bit even as they happened. He also noticed that he could recognize and allow his feelings of anxiety to exist in his body, even as he recognized and allowed the thoughts driven by the anxiety to arise and pass away.

As he became less reactive to the self-perpetuating cycles of anxiety and thinking, Bill also learned to recognize and to let go of much of his harsh self-criticism. He saw even those judgments as just another set of thoughts, rather than being a true statement of who he was. Bill's ability to observe his thoughts and let them go, and suspend any negative self-image as a result of these thoughts, allowed him to cope with his feelings of anxiety in a more calm and controlled manner. Bill's mindfulness practice has taught him to manage his anxiety by not engaging and remaining nonjudgmental.

Ellen's Story

Ellen wakes in the middle of the night with her heart racing, a feeling of choking, in a sweat, and with thoughts about immediate death filling her head. She is having a panic attack. It has been happening for over three years now. She has noticed that the panic attacks come more often if she is "stressed out." Just this morning, Ellen confided to a coworker that she has just ended a relationship of almost two years, and feels "really stressed out." As the attack unfolds, Ellen feels worse and worse. "I hate these attacks," she thinks. "This feels like the last one, maybe worse. I think I am going to die."

Then Ellen recalls the lessons of her mindfulness meditation class. The teacher emphasized seeing things as if they are here for the first time. She called this way of approaching things with a *beginner's mind*. Ellen tries to relate to her experience of this panic attack that way—with a beginner's mind. She begins to pay closer attention to her body sensations, and to her breathing, and then to the thoughts she is having. She begins to observe them and to allow them to exist, without judgments. It is not easy, but she persists. She repeatedly returns her focus to the sensations of her breath, as it flows in and out. With this steady focus, she then opens her attention to include everything else that is happening.

She begins to feel some distance between herself and the panic attacks. She does not become so fixed upon the thoughts, or on how bad things seem to be. She recognizes that the frightening thoughts may not even be true. And, that she is not her thoughts. After a time, things cool down. Ellen notices that only a few minutes have passed and that already she feels better. She realizes this attack is almost over at a time when the earlier ones were just getting started. She feels a bit of hope and some confidence in her own ability to work with the panic if it comes back. Truly, she thinks, each experience *is* different. Ellen's nonjudgmental approach allows her not to participate in the panic attacks. Her mindfulness practice has allowed her not to become engulfed by the anxiety.

Mindfulness Exercises

Everyone falls unconsciously into old habits of mind and body, of attention and inattention, which result in not being present for one's own life. The consequences of this inattention can be quite costly in that each of us may be missing out on events and relationships, ignoring important information and messages about our own life, and even possibly compromising our own health.

An important antidote to this tendency to "tune-out," or go on "automatic pilot," is to practice *mindfulness*. Everyone has the capacity for mindfulness. To develop that capacity, or to practice mindfulness, means to pay more careful attention, moment-by-moment. Mindfulness is an awareness that arises when one connects and pays attention carefully, in a nonjudging and allowing way, to whatever experience is arising here, in the present moment. The domain of mindfulness, the field for one's attention, includes what is going on inside one's skin, as well as what is happening on the outside. Throughout life, through whichever sense gate life appears—eyes, ears, nose, tongue, body—mindfulness is the awareness that knows and recognizes seeing, hearing, smelling, tasting, feeling, or thinking. Those experiences are happening in this present moment.

So, mindfulness practice is not about thinking at all. It is about attention and the awareness that recognizes thinking, and all other sense experiences. To practice mindfulness, one has to establish attention in the present moment, and allow what is happening to happen, maintain contact, and observe it. This is sometimes called practicing *being, not doing*. Simply being with what is happening, yet maintaining conscious contact is the key. Paying attention with interest and friendliness and avoiding the need to change anything or to make anything happen is mindfulness. Learning to practice mindfulness in this way *is* to practice meditation. One should learn to rest in the inherent quality of being, sensitive and aware, in each moment, as life unfolds. If one can practice "being," and become more present and more aware *of* one's life, this will lead to being more present *in* that life. The "doing" engages in the will to be more informed, more responsive, and less driven by habits of reaction and inattention.

Steps for Practicing Mindfulness

Step 1. Use the sensation of breath as an anchor for attention and awareness in the present moment. Mindfulness is an awareness that arises when one pays attention in a nonjudging way. For many people, it is easy to take a narrow focus on one object, like breath sensations, to develop mindfulness. *Mindfulness is not only about the breath, but one can choose the breath as an object because it is always there with one.*

Step 2. Establish attention on the single focus of the breath sensation, wherever the breath feels most easily as it comes and goes in one's body. Don't try to control breath, or to make anything happen. Simply let the breath come and go. Bring as much and as continuous attention to the cycle of the breath: in, pause, out, pause, in, pause, out, pause, in, pause, out, pause, and on and on.

Step 3. After establishing attention on the breath sensation, widen the focus to include awareness of all body sensations as well as the breath. Simply allow the sensations to happen as each breath passes. The focus now is on the strongest or clearest sensation. Notice how they change, and how one follows another.

Step 4. After a while widen the focus again. Include all that is present. This means all sounds, sights, tastes, smells, thoughts, and emotions. Practice applying a friendly and welcoming attitude to whatever arises, allowing it to happen while remaining in conscious contact (mindful) and being present with it. Practice being with the entire range of unfolding experiences as continuously and consciously as possible—aware of each event as it arises, changes, and then fades. Relax, observe, and allow each experience to be just as it is.

Step 5. Anytime the mind wanders, or there are feelings of being lost, confused, discouraged, or frustrated, notice these feelings. Be kind and patient with them. If there are feelings of distraction, gently narrow the focus of attention again to the breath sensation. Do this as many times as necessary. It is okay. Everyone has a wandering mind. The most important thing is the quality of awareness in each moment. One moment of mindfulness, one breath, can be quite profound.

Hints for Practicing Mindfulness in Daily Life

1. *Expect the mind to wander.* Practice kindness and patience when this happens, and gently return awareness to the breath sensation.
2. *Notice any tendency to be "hard on yourself."* Beware of being critical when the attention wanders, notice frustration about that, and recognize that nothing has been done wrong. See such criticisms and judgments as just another form of thinking, and let them go.
3. *Expect to feel some relaxation.* A calming of mind and body is a normal reaction. This relaxed feeling is an ally, but not the ultimate goal of mindfulness practice. Relaxation helps to be more present and mindful. Being present with awareness is easier when mind and body are calmed and relaxed.
4. *Expect to become more mindful with practice.* Expect to notice more things, including more painful things. This is progress. When there is pain, try to hold the situation with compassion and kindness, and remain in contact with it. Allow the experience to continue to unfold, maintain sensitive and nonjudgmental feelings. Working with the pain or painful experiences this way

trains one to remain open in all sorts of situations, and to the possibilities there.

5. *This staying with pain takes some faith and courage as well.* Have faith that one is not damaged or destroyed by contact with the painful or unpleasant. Have courage to stay in contact and present with awareness in the midst of discomfort and fear. When staying present with the unpleasant and painful, one discovers that mindfulness is not tarnished or damaged.

6. *Finally, do not try too hard when practicing mindfulness.* Be authentic. Do not try to make anything special happen, or try to attain any special states or effects. Simply relax, and pay attention as closely and as sensitively as possible to what is present now. Experience life just as it is, with open attention.

CONCLUSION

Meditation practices have existed since ancient times and in diverse cultures. These practices have historically been the vehicles for profound personal healing and transformation. They are understood only through direct personal experience and practice, usually with the guidance of an experienced teacher. Mindfulness is an awareness that is available to all human beings, and can be cultivated and realized through meditation practice.

In the past few decades, Western medicine and psychology have taken an increased interest in the therapeutic benefits of different meditation practices including mindfulness meditation. There are now growing numbers of reports which suggest that meditation practice can have a positive impact on a variety of physical and psychological conditions. Clinicians have developed specific meditation-based interventions to aid clinical populations suffering from a range of conditions from stress to chronic pain to disturbances of mood to dysfunctional behaviors.

Since the research on meditation is still in its early stages, important considerations and directions for research require more rigorous study of different practices and the variables involved. As the application and understanding of mindfulness grows, healers in contemporary Western culture can join with their kin from other times and places in realizing the transforming power of being present.

REFERENCES

Baer, R. (2003). Mindfulness training as a clinical intervention: A conceptual and empirical review. *Clinical Psychology: Science and Practice, 10*(2), 125-143.

Benson, H. (1993). The relaxation response. In D. Goleman and J. Gurin (Eds.). *Mind body medicine: How to use your mind for better health* (pp. 233-257). Yonkers, NY: Consumer Reports Books.

Boorstein, S. (1996). Clinical applications of meditation. In B.N. Scotton, A.B. Chinen, & J.R. Battista (Eds.), *Textbook of transpersonal psychiatry and psychology* (pp. 344-354). New York: Basic Books.

Brach, T. (2003). *Radical acceptance: Embracing your life with the heart of Buddha.* New York: Bantam Books.

Epstein, M. (1996). *Thoughts without a thinker: Psychotherapy from a Buddhist perspective.* New York: Basic Books, a division of HarperCollins.

Feldman, Christina. (1998). *Thorsons principles of meditation.* London: Thorsons.

Goenka, S.N. (2005). Vipassana meditation: the technique. Retrieved February 7, 2007, from http://www.dharma.org/en/vipassana.shtml.

Goldenberg, D.L., Kaplan, K.N., & Nadeau, M.G. (1994). A controlled study of a stress reduction, cognitive-behavioral treatment program in fibromyalgia. *Musculoskeletal Pain, 2,* 53-66.

Goleman, D. (1977). *Varieties of the meditative experience.* New York: E.P. Dutton.

Gunaratana, H. (1992). *Mindfulness in plain English.* Boston: Wisdom Publications.

Hanh, Thich Nhat. (1999). *The heart of the Buddha's teaching.* New York: Broadway.

Hayes, S.C., Follette, V., & Linehan, M. (Eds.). (2004). *Mindfulness and acceptance.* New York: Guilford Press.

Hayes, S.C., Strosahl, K., & Wilson, K.G. (1999). *Acceptance and commitment therapy.* New York: Guilford Press.

Ingram, R.E., Miranda, J., & Segal, Z.V. (1998). *Cognitive vulnerability to depression.* New York: Guilford Press.

Judd, L.L., Akiskal, H.S., & Paulus, M.D. (1997). The role and clinical significance of subsyndromal depressive symptoms (SDD) in unipolar major depressive disorder. *Journal of Affective Disorders, 45*(1-2), 5-18.

Kabat-Zinn, J. (1982). An outpatient program in behavioral medicine for chronic pain in patients based on the practice of mindfulness meditation: Theoretical considerations and preliminary results. *General Hospital Psychiatry, 4,* 33-47.

Kabat-Zinn, J. (2003). Mindfulness-based interventions in context: Past, present, and future. *Clinical Psychology: Science and Practice, 10*(2), 144-156.

Kabat-Zinn, J., Lipworth, L., & Burney, R. (1985). The clinical use of mindfulness meditation for the self-regulation of chronic pain. *Journal of Behavioral Medicine, 8,* 163-190.

Kabat-Zinn, J., Lipworth, L., Burney, R., & Sellers, W. (1986). Four year follow-up of a meditation-based program for the self-regulation of chronic pain: Treatment outcomes and compliance. *Clinical Journal of Pain, 2,* 159-173.

Kabat-Zinn, J., Massion, A.O., Kristeller, J., Peterson, L.G., Fletcher, K.E., Pbert, L., et al. (1992). Effectiveness of a meditation-based stress reduction program in the treatment of anxiety disorders. *American Journal of Psychiatry, 149,* 936-943.

Kabat-Zinn, J., Wheeler, E., Light, T., Skillings, A., Scharf, M., Cropley, T.G., et al. (1998). Influence of a mindfulness-based stress reduction intervention on rates of skin clearing in patients with moderate to severe psoriasis undergoing phototherapy (UVB) and photochemotherapy (PUVA). *Psychosomatic Medicine, 60,* 625-632.

Kaplan, K.H., Goldenberg, D.L., & Galvin-Nadeau, M. (1993). The impact of a meditation-based stress reduction program on fibromyalgia. *General Hospital Psychiatry, 15,* 284-289.

Kristeller, J.L. & Hallett, C.B. (1999). An exploratory study of a meditation-based intervention for binge-eating disorder. *Journal of Health Psychology, 4,* 357-363.

Lao-tsu. (1988). *Tao te ching,* translated by S. Mitchell. New York: Harper Perrennial.

Linehan, M. (1993a). *Cognitive-behavioral treatment of borderline personality disorder.* New York: Guilford Press.

Linehan, M. (1993b). *Skills training manual for treating borderline personality disorder.* New York: Guilford Press.

Marlatt, G.A. (1994). Addiction, mindfulness, and acceptance. In S.C. Hayes, N.S. Jacobson, V.M. Follette, & M.J. Dougher (Eds.), *Acceptance and change: Content and context in psychotherapy* (pp. 175-197). Reno, NV: Context Press.

Marlatt, G.A. (2002). *Buddhist philosophy and the treatment of addictive behavior. Cognitive and Behavioral Practice, 9,* 44-49.

Merriam-Webster's Dictionary (1997). Springfield, MA: Merriam-Webster, Inc.

National Institute of Health (2004). *Mind-body medicine: An overview.* Retrieved March 30, 2007, from http:/nccam.nih.gov/health/backgrounds/mindbody.htm.

Reibel, D., Greeson, J., Brainard, G., & Rosenzweig, S. (2001). Mindfulness-based stress reduction and health-related quality of life in a heterogeneous patient population. *General Hospital Psychiatry, 23,* 183-192.

Rosenberg, Larry & David Guy. (1998). *Breath by breath.* Boston: Shambhala.

Schuhmacher, S. & Woerner, G. (Eds.). (1994). *The Encyclopedia of Eastern Philosophy & Religion.* Shambhala Publications.

Scotton, B. (1996). Introduction and definitions of transpersonal psychiatry. In B.N. Scotton, A.B. Chinen, & J.R. Battista (Eds.), *Textbook of transpersonal psychiatry and psychology* (pp. 3-8). New York: Basic Books.

Segal, Z.V., Williams, J.M.G., & Teasdale, J.D. (2002). *Mindfulness-based cognitive therapy for depression: A new approach to preventing relapse.* New York: Guilford Press.

Shapiro, S.L., Schwartz, G.E., & Bonner, G. (1998). Effects of mindfulness-based stress reduction on medical and premedical students. *Journal of Behavioral Medicine, 21,* 581-599.

Smith, J. (Ed.). (1999). *Radiant mind: Essential Buddhist teachings and texts.* New York: Riverhead Books.

Speca, M., Carlson, L.E., Goodey, E., & Angen, M. (2000). A randomized, wait-list controlled clinical trial: The effect of a mindfulness meditation-based stress reduction program on mood and symptoms of stress in cancer outpatients. *Psychosomatic Medicine, 62,* 613-622.

Tacon, A.M., McComb, J., Caldera, Y., & Randolph, P. (2003). Mindfulness meditation, anxiety reduction, and heart disease. *Family Community Health, 26,* 25-33.

Taylor, E. (1997). Introduction. In M. Murphy & S. Donovan (Eds.), *The physical and psychological effects of meditation: A review of contemporary research with a comprehensive bibliography 1931-1996* (2nd ed.) (pp. 1-32). Sausalito, CA: Institute of Noetic Sciences.

Teasdale, J.D., Segal, Z.V., & Williams, M.G. (1995). How does cognitive therapy prevent depressive relapse and why should attentional control (mindfulness training) help? *Behaviour Research and Therapy, 33,* 25-39.

Teasdale, J.D., Segal, Z.V., Williams, M.G., Ridgeway, V.A., Soulsby, J.M., & Lau, M.A. (2000). Prevention of relapse/recurrence in major depression by mindfulness-based cognitive therapy. *Journal of Consulting and Clinical Psychology, 68,* 615-623.

Watts, A. (1961). Psychotherapy east and west. New York: Random House.

Weissbecker, I., Salmon, P., Studts, J., Floyd, A., Dedert, E., & Sephton, S. (2002). Mindfulness-based stress reduction and sense of coherence among women with fibromyalgia. *Journal of Clinical Psychology in Medical Settings, 9,* 297-307.

Chapter 3

Spirituality

Mary P. Van Hook

A walk in the woods, a time for meditation, a prayer, candles lit in memory or celebration, a time listening to music, a moment of silence, a personal journal, a sweat lodge ceremony, a view of a sunset, the sacrament of reconciliation—spirituality assumes many external forms in the lives of people. Social workers and other helping professionals are increasingly recognizing the value of including spirituality and the related concept of religion as part of a holistic approach to understanding and working with people (ben Asher, 2001; Canda & Furman, 1999; Cascio, 1998; Dossey & Dossey, 1998; Jacobs, 1997; Koenig, 1999; Van Hook, Hugen, & Aguilar, 2001).

In the context of this chapter spirituality is regarded as "not one dimension among many in life; rather, it permeates and gives meaning to life" (Moberg, 2001b, p. 15). Canda and Furman (1999) assign spirituality a vital role in the helping process. They describe "spirituality as the heart of helping—the heart of empathy and care, the pulse of compassion, the vital flow of practice wisdom, and the driving force of action for service" (Canda & Furman, 1999, p. xv). The incorporation of spirituality into the healing process does not represent a specific treatment technique, but instead is a recognition that spirituality can play a vital role in the healing process and that it is important to find appropriate ways to support this particular aspect of healing. Spirituality as part of the therapeutic process opens the door to an important realm of human existence and taps the strengths and issues that are present within the individual.

Introduction to Alternative and Complementary Therapies
© 2008 by The Haworth Press, Taylor & Francis Group. All rights reserved.
doi:10.1300/5987_03

Despite recent interest in the role of spirituality/religion in the lives of people and its role in helping professionals, many therapists feel uncertain about effective and appropriate ways in which to include these dimensions in the therapeutic process. The tradition of separation between spirituality/religion and counseling within social work and other mental health fields has left many counselors skeptical and uncertain about the role of spirituality/religion within counseling. It has also left them without an understanding of ways to draw upon spirituality as a means of healing in the lives of individuals and families (ben Asher, 2001; Canda & Furman, 1999; Frame, 2003; Hugen, 2001; Walsh, 1998). A national study conducted in 1997, for example, revealed that 73 percent of social workers reported they did not receive any instruction in these related topics during their social work education (Canda & Furman, 1999). In addition to lack of training, Canda and Furman (1999) also indicate that as a result of this tradition of separation, "sometimes students and practitioners are criticized by instructors even for broaching the subject" (p. xvi).

Reflecting a shift in this divide, in recognition of the important role that spirituality and religion frequently play in the lives of people, social work and other mental health professionals have recognized the importance of professional counselors to be culturally competent in the areas of spirituality and religion and have come to incorporate content in these areas in their professional education. Fortunately, there is a growing body of literature designed to help practitioners to understand spirituality and incorporate it into their practice.

The purpose of this chapter is not to equip mental health professionals to become spiritual counselors but instead to enable them to help their clients draw upon spiritual strengths in the healing process and identify barriers that would prevent clients from accessing their spirituality. The role of counselor is to focus upon ways to use spirituality in a collaborative relationship with the client, thus enabling that client to address problems and life experiences within a spiritual context. Spirituality is seen therefore as a resource for promoting the client's efforts to resolve or cope with problems. This model of practice involves an understanding of the role of spirituality in the lives of clients as well as how cultural and religious traditions impact spirituality and developmental issues which impinge on spirituality. As is necessary in other therapeutic approaches, it is critical that counselors engage in self-reflection regarding the role of religion and spirituality in their own lives (Canda & Furman, 1999; Frame, 2003; Hugen, 2001; Sherwood, 2002). Spirituality as part of the therapeutic approach can be incorporated into those counseling models that are based on a strengths perspective and recognize the role of life stories in therapy and the interactive process by which individuals construct their meaning systems based on life events which in turn influence how these events are experienced.

Before discussing the place of spirituality in practice, it is important to understand the concept of healing because incorporating spirituality into therapy reflects the tradition of healing. Walsh (1999), in her classic book *Spiritual Resources in Family Therapy*, distinguishes between healing and treatment. Healing is described as "a therapeutic relationship that encourages clients' own inherent healing potential . . . Healing involves a gathering of resources within the person, the family, and the community, and is fostered through the therapeutic relationship" (p. 33). Healing is the process of becoming whole. It contrasts with treatment where the emphasis is upon the action of an external agent.

As Walsh describes it, healing can occur on many levels—physically, emotionally, interpersonally, and spiritually. People can heal emotionally from events that cannot be cured physically or improved economically. Although traumatic events cannot be erased from the lives and memories of people, the pain and emotional injuries of such events can be healed. The concept of healing is very important for social workers and other counselors for although they can sometimes help people resolve a problem, there are other situations in which individuals must learn to either live with their problem, or to endure, adapt to, or cope with it. Mental health professionals frequently work with individuals who are facing situations that require endurance or adaptation and are struggling to find new meanings to life events. In hospice programs, for example, counselors regularly help individuals and family members face the inevitability of death. People seek help through therapy for the wounds of childhood physical or sexual abuse that are impairing their adult lives. Individuals must resume their lives after the betrayal of a marital partner. Even when people are facing problems that must be addressed by action, issues of meaning also emerge, as in the case of parents coping with a child born with developmental disabilities, or an individual whose partner needs care, or someone whose economic problems are due to the loss of a job or business. Suffering is part of the human journey and often prompts within the individual questions of meaning and other spiritual concerns which those in the helping profession may be called upon to address. As discussed subsequently in this chapter, it is in the areas of emotional and interpersonal meaning that spirituality can contribute to healing. Further, there is growing evidence that spirituality can also contribute to physical health. The concept of healing is especially compatible with the role of spirituality because both healing and spirituality stress the role of marshalling the resources of individuals and the powerful role that spirituality can play in influencing the meaning systems that can promote the healing process.

SPIRITUALITY AND RELIGION

Although spirituality has been described in many different ways, some basic themes are present. Canda describes the spiritual aspect of the self as relating to the "person's search for meaning and morally fulfilling relationships between oneself, other people, and encompassing universe, and the ontological ground of existence, whether a person understands this in terms that are theistic, atheistic, nontheistic, or any combination of these" (Canda & Furman, 1999, p. 44). Canda and Furman (1999) summarize the concepts inherent in spirituality as follows. Spirituality "is understood as an essential or holistic quality of the human being that cannot be reduced to any part of a person" (p. 44). It is "an aspect of the person concerned with the development of meaning and morality and relationship with a divine or ultimate reality" (p. 44). It can "also include transpersonal experiences in which consciousness transcends the ordinary limits of ego and boundary boundaries, such as mystical experiences" (Canda & Furman, 1999, p. 44). According to Watkins (2001),

> (spirituality) includes the inner resources and ultimate concern of older persons. It provides the basic value around which all other values are evaluated; the person's central philosophy of life—religious, nonreligious, and antireligious—that provides direction for their attitudes and behavior. (p. 134)

As is evident from these definitions, spirituality plays a critical role in the meanings attributed to life events and to people's self-identity and their relationships with others.

Although for some individuals spirituality is experienced apart from religion, for many others spirituality is set within the context of their religious experience. The vast majority of people in the United States describe themselves as believing in a God or a universal spirit and indicate that they pray on a regular basis (Hugen, 2001). Spirituality for these individuals is experienced frequently within a religious context and is an essential part of their religious life. Religious traditions shape the meaning and experience of their spirituality. Religion is understood to include "the patterning of spiritual beliefs and practices into social institutions, with community support and traditions maintained over time" (Canda, 1997, p. 173). Each religion has cultural, historical and organizational dimensions as well a set of beliefs and an experiential component. Religious groups and personal experience shape the sense of spirituality of many people. It is thus important to understand how religious traditions influence the worldview of people within specific groups and to be familiar with the potential spiritual resources and issues present within each group.

The diversity of religious traditions even within the United States is enormous and continues to grow as people from different parts of the world bring their religious traditions with them (Hugen, 2001). Mosques and Buddhist and Hindu temples have taken their place as part of the American landscape along side Catholic, Orthodox, and Protestant churches, and Jewish synagogues. Religious institutions with signs in Spanish, Korean, Chinese, Vietnamese, Creole, Arabic, and many other languages are found in rural as well as urban communities. Such religious diversity requires social workers to seek to understand different religious traditions as part of their expertise in cultural diversity.

The societal and organizational aspects of religion also make it important to understand how cultural and historical aspects influence religion. Members of the First Nations experienced oppression and accompanying efforts to extinguish their religious practices that had strengthened the people. Because of the punishment meted out to people who practiced their traditional religion and owing to the pressure to become Christian, some of their traditional beliefs and practices were cloaked in terms of Christianity. The boarding school experience in which young people were forcibly removed from their families, culture, and religion and typically placed within a Christian setting also influenced religious practices. Some of these experiences resulted in a blending of traditional religion and Christian practices (Brave Heart, 2001). Brave Heart (2001) describes several ways in which this has occurred. The sacred spiritual link between the Lakota Nation and the Buffalo Nation was lost with the destruction of the buffalo and the loss of land. This combination is identified as an ongoing source of trauma and grief for the Lakota (Brave Heart, 2001). She also describes how oppression has led to a sense of historical trauma as well as the devaluing of women who were once viewed as sacred and of sex which was considered a sacred act "through which the spirits were connected" (Brave Heart, 2001, p. 21). Acts of violence in the United States and other countries that have been perpetrated by members of the Islamic faith have led to discussions of whether Islam is a religion that promotes violence toward others or promotes love and justice. Repressive policies toward women by the Taliban in Afghanistan and other Mideastern countries have raised the issue of whether Islam is a faith that represses women or affirms the worth and dignity of women. Catholicism is experienced differently by members of a variety of ethnic groups including those individuals who are Polish (Folwarski & Marganoff, 1996), Irish (McGolderick, 1996), Italian (Giordano & McGolderick, 1996), or Puerto Rican (Garcia-Preto, 1996; Canda & Furman, 1999). Aguilar (2001) describes ways in which the history of oppression experienced by Mexican Americans has influenced their expression of Catholicism. Mexican Americans who lived in communities in which they were a minority felt unwelcome and discriminated against by the American Catholics. As a result, participation in the organizational life of the church was not viewed as important and this historical context still lives in the memories and religious lives of families. In contrast, individuals who lived in communities in which Hispanics were the majority became invested in the parish life of the church (Aguilar, 2001). Members of Hispanic groups are assuming an even larger proportion of Catholic and Protestant groups within the United States and bring their unique traditions and history with them (Canda & Furman, 1999). Grant (2001) portrays the interaction between the history of oppression and the meaning of religion for African Americans. In the context of oppression, African Americans found in the church and their religion a source of refuge, affirmation, and mutual support. Immigrants from different nations bring to the United States their traditional worship practices and codes of behavior.

WHY SHOULD SPIRITUALITY AND RELIGION BE INCLUDED IN THE COUNSELING PROCESS?

It is important to find ways to incorporate spirituality and religion in the counseling process and to move beyond some of the separation that in the past has impeded this process. The client's perspectives on life and the identification of the client's spiritual and related resources should be incorporated into the counseling process. To ask about spirituality is strength-based and demonstrates respect for the client's right to self-determination. In fact, to avoid discussing spirituality when it is important to the client conveys a message that what the client wants to talk about is not valid (Watkins, 2001), and thus the therapist fails to provide a holistic approach to the therapeutic process.

Impetus for Incorporating Spirituality

The impetus for opening the door to spirituality, for finding ways to incorporate spirituality and possible associated religious traditions comes from a variety of sources. First, those counseling models which stress the meaning of systems in the lives of individuals and families including spirituality and religion require counselors to understand the paradigms that shape how clients view their world, current problems, and possible solutions to their problems. Narrative therapy, for example, refers to therapists as coeditors and stresses the importance of developing stories that build on strengths and solutions rather than those that are problem saturated (White & Epston, 1990). Social constructionist perspectives with their concept of knowledge as created require us to have a respectful and deep understanding of the impact of how people view their world in the therapeutic process (Thayne, 1998). Strength-based approaches to therapy emphasize the importance of looking for sources of strength within the lives of clients (Seeleby, 1992).

Second, there is a growing recognition by health professionals that spirituality and religion play important roles in the lives of people from a wide variety of cultural backgrounds (Canda & Furman, 1999; Frame, 2003; Van Hook et al., 2001). The dramatic success of the recent movie *The Passion* (Gibson, 2004), depicting the last hours of Jesus Christ surprised the entertainment industry as it revealed the strong interest in religion in current American society. Religion has been recognized as a potent force for goodness or tragedy. The compassionate work of Mother Theresa and her order of the Sisters of Charity or the Dalai Lama can be contrasted with the horror of Jonestown or the suffering caused by some Islamic radicals who have perpetrated violence on thousands throughout the world in the name of their faith. Fellow members of the Islamic faith have in turn become victims of hate crimes.

Third, a growing body of literature points out the positive role that spirituality and more specifically religion can play in promoting both mental and physical health (Cummings, Neff, & Husaini, 2003; Koenig, 1999; Moberg, 2001b; Pargament, 1997; Parker et al., 2003; Van Hook & Aguliar, 2001), while recognizing that deeply spiritual and religious people can become seriously ill. Research regarding the impact of spirituality and religion is complicated because no single measure can adequately address either of these aspects of life. It is always important to identify how each study defines spirituality or religion (Moberg, 2001c). Some of the following studies relate to spirituality in a more general sense of the term while others address spirituality as embedded within a religious tradition as well as other aspects of religion.

Spirituality and religion appear to promote health in a variety of ways, including health promotion behaviors, meaning systems, hope, a sense of community (belonging), and beliefs and practices that enable people to address the circumstances in their lives that contribute to distress and disease (Perry, 1998). Healthy lifestyles help to promote health and these lifestyles are encouraged through the spiritual views held by many religious traditions that grant dignity to the body. Christian groups have traditionally described the body as the "Temple of God" (Perry, 1998). Seventh Day Adventists endorse this view along with the belief that healthy living prepares them for heaven (Vander Waal & McMullin, 2001). Mormons believe in an inseparable link between the body, the mind, and the spirit and thus maintaining good physical health enhances mental and spiritual health (Haynes, 2001). The latter two groups have developed extensive dietary and life style prescriptions that support healthy lifestyles and have resulted in improved health indices. The Lakota tradition believes that the body is a container for the spirit, a gift from the Creator (Brave Heart, 2001). Hindus view God as present in the bodies of human beings as well as other creatures (Singh, 2001). Buddhists regard the body as a precious vehicle for seeking enlightenment and helping others (Canda, 2001).

People who hold religious beliefs and participate in the organized life of a religious tradition are generally less likely to abuse alcohol and drugs and to experience the related health problems. This is especially true for women and adolescents (Booth & Martin, 1998; Donahue & Benson, 1995; Moberg, 2001d). This pattern can be explained in various ways, including experiencing the love of God that can reduce the need for mind altering chemicals, holding beliefs that support abstinence or prohibit abuse of substances, and being part of a social support system that provides a sense of belonging and reinforces nondrinking behavior (Booth & Martin, 1998).

Prayer, an important spiritual ritual in a wide variety of religious traditions, appears to play a role in supporting health. In several studies, prayer either by others or by the ill person was associated with improved health outcomes (Moberg, 2001b).

Studies with older adults generally show that religiosity and spirituality are associated with lower levels of anxiety about death, less alcoholism, fewer suicides, better marriages, greater adaptation to Alzheimer's disease care taking, reduced loneliness, hopefulness among disabled older adults, and general mental health (Koenig, George, & Titus, 2004; Moberg, 2001a). Moberg (2001a) found that among elderly African-American women living in poverty, faith in God was a way of coping with hardship and enhancing their self-esteem. Their relationship with God enabled them to believe that their hardship was part of a divine plan and that they would be rewarded either in this life or in the next. Spirituality associated with religion has been associated with decreased depression in older adults (Cummings et al., 2003; Koenig, 1994; Parker et al., 2003; Roff et al., 2004). In a recent study with older adults living in the community, turning to God for a relationship, seeking God's care, and asking for forgiveness emerged as important coping strategies in dealing with the difficult transition typical of the older years (Van Hook & Rivera, 2004). In terms of religious involvement, the strongest effects were for people with a deep personal religious faith who live out their faith by active involvement in their religious congregations (Koenig, 2000).

A fourth reason for including spirituality in the counseling process is that spirituality has been identified as promoting resiliency (the process by which people manage not only to endure hardships but also to create and sustain lives that have meaning and contribute to those around them). In Werner's ground breaking longitudinal study of Hawaiian youth who had experienced major risk factors, spirituality was one of the factors that contributed to resiliency among young adults. Spirituality emerged in terms of a spiritual meaning in life and religious connections with a church or religious community (Werner & Smith, 1992). A small qualitative study conducted with African Americans who had "made it against the odds" (Gordon & Song, 1994) revealed that spiritual connections were included in factors that promoted resiliency.

Walsh (1998) identifies spirituality as one of the important resources for resiliency in families. "Personal faith supports the belief that we can overcome our challenges" (p. 71). She describes a transcendent value system as one that enables us to define our lives as meaningful and significant. She sees spirituality as a link to the transcendent (Walsh, 1998). Religion and spirituality can also promote resiliency by offering a sense of meaning in the context of difficult times. Wright (1999) describes the medium of therapeutic conversations about beliefs regarding spirituality and religion as an effective way to create understanding that makes the creation of changes and healing with families possible.

Shadow Side

Yet all powerful resources can also have shadow sides. While spiritual and religious support can offer hope, it can also impede coping and mastery, foster an inability to invest life with meaning, and create distress depending on the problems people face (Van Hook et al., 2001; Walsh, 1998; Pargament, 1997).

An individual who contracts HIV through a homosexual relationship could find it difficult to seek help from a religious community that condemns such relationships. A person whose depression makes her or him feel alienated from God could feel burdened by additional guilt. People with perfectionist concepts of what is expected of them by the spiritual tradition can feel cut-off when he or she has failed to meet these standards. As discussed subsequently in terms of assessment, one of the steps of the counselor is to identify with clients what role their spiritual and religious beliefs are playing at this point in time.

ETHICAL ISSUES

Canda and Furman (1999) identify a code of ethics of spiritually sensitive social work practice that articulates the Social Work Code of Ethics in a spiritual context. While the following discussion is tied specifically to the profession of social work code of ethics, many of these basic principles are important to mental health professions in general. The following section identifies the core social work value and the related ethical principles of the NASW code of ethics. The statement following each principle briefly summarizes the nature of spiritually sensitive practice in terms of this tenet of the Code of Ethics as developed by Canda and Furman (1999).

"Value: Service. Ethical Principle: Social workers' primary goal is to help people in need and to address social problems." "Spiritually sensitive social workers elevate service to others above self-interest" . . . and recognize that such service "promotes the growth of both worker and client." (pp. 30, 31)

"Value: Social Justice. Ethical principle: Social workers challenge social injustice." "Spiritually sensitive social workers pursue social change" to promote social justice with and for persons and their eco systems. (p. 31)

"Value: Dignity and worth of the person. Ethical principle: Social workers respect the inherent dignity and worth of the person." Spiritually sensitive social workers treat each person with care," respectful of individual differences. (p. 32)

"Value: Importance of Human Relationships. Ethical principle: Social Workers recognize the central importance of human relationships." Spiritually sensitive social workers understand the value of human relationships and seek to strengthen them. (p. 32)

"Value: Integrity. Ethical Principle: Social workers behave in a trustworthy manner." Spiritually sensitive social workers seek to carryout the mission and values of their profession. (p. 33)

"Value: Competence. Ethical Principle: Social workers practice within their areas of competence and develop and enhance their professional expertise." Social workers seek to enhance their competence, including the spiritual life of clients, and to contribute to the knowledge of the profession. (p. 34)

A more complete description of the nature of spiritually sensitive social work practice is contained in Canda and Furman (1999, pp. 30-34).

SPIRITUALITY AND COUNSELING

Bullis (1996) contrasts a spiritual model of practice with the medical model. The spiritual model incorporates the metaphysical and transcendent aspects of the person as well as the physical, emotional, and intellectual that are part of the medical model. The spiritual model is described as enabling counselors to be more holistic in their approach to healing. The following section describes ways to incorporate spirituality into the assessment process, life cycle issues, and treatment approaches that can address spirituality.

Assessment of Spirituality

Before discussing specific ways to assess spirituality and/or religion in the lives of people, it is important to recognize that this process belongs to the arena of "knowing" rather than mere "information." Knowing pushes beyond a set of facts to the meaning of these facts in the life of another person which creates a sense of understanding. For example, a statement on a face sheet of an agency that someone is Catholic or Hindu is not the same as a series of questions that relate to the meaning of this religion in the life of the person and how this meaning in turn relates possibly to the current situation. If a family member is dying, issues related to important rituals prior to and following death or interpretations of the possibility and nature of life after death become extremely relevant in the "knowing" process.

The process of assessing spiritual issues reflects the complex nature of spirituality and its possible religious context. Social workers and members of other professional groups can use several specific techniques as well as incorporate this important topic within their general assessment interview process.

Because assessment is a reciprocal process, our clients are also assessing us in terms of the areas that we discuss comfortably, our values, and our ability to understand them as individuals. Since spirituality and religion are often deeply meaningful issues, clients may be hesitant to trust the counselor if they do not believe that their concerns will be treated with honor and respect (Hodge, 2003b). Demonstrating interest in and respect for the dimension of the spiritual in the lives of our clients will facilitate the process of being able to identify and use the spiritual resources.

David Hodge (2003b) suggests that qualitative measures are especially effective in the area of spirituality and religion in counseling. He has written a useful handbook, *Spiritual Assessment: A Handbook for Helping Professionals,* to help clinicians use assessment tools to explore the spiritual lives of clients.

Therapeutic Conversation

The therapeutic conversation is an assessment approach through which the counselor opens the door to spirituality and religion in the life of the client, especially as it relates to the issue at hand. Hodge (2003a,b) describes the therapeutic conversation as a "spiritual anthropology." This conversation can include a variety of dimensions—the spiritual and religious support system and how it is experienced, relevant beliefs that impact the current life event, nature of the relationship to the divine, religious prescriptions that influence the current situation, the moral compass of life, the emotional aspect of spirituality and religion, and important rituals. Such a directed conversation can identify how clients interpret life issues within their social context. Spiritual and religious traditions influence views of illness, along with potential sources of healing and support. A Christian scientist family's interpretation of physical illness in the spiritual-mind realm would certainly differ from that of a Catholic or Protestant family that recognizes and supports the use of health professionals. People also sometimes view illness as punishment. As a result, people with HIV/AIDS have sometimes been reluctant to seek help from members of their religious community due to the stigma involved. Views of marriage also play important roles. A woman struggling with whether or not she should leave an abusive spouse can be influenced by the beliefs of her religious tradition regarding the sanctity and permanence of marriage. However, the same woman might experience the full support of her religious community if her husband should die. Religious and spiritual traditions have profoundly different views regarding death and the nature of life after death. Understanding these beliefs and practices can be important for counselors working with families addressing a terminal illness or the loss of a family member through death. Spiritual traditions shape the specific meaning of suffering (Van Hook & Aguilar, 2001).

These directed therapeutic conversations can identify resources present within the spiritual and/or religious tradition of the client, such as caring and community supports of food and financial help or support for emotional needs during times of suffering. Religious traditions and spirituality may lend support for individuals in the areas of emotional connection and a sense of purpose and meaning. People may feel worthwhile when seeing themselves as children of God or when sensing that the divine exists within each individual. They may be strengthened by the belief that they can turn to a divine being as a partner in dealing with difficult times. Research has shown that during painful times such coping efforts are associated with improved mental health and more favorable outcomes (Koenig, 1999; Levin & Chatters, 1998; Pargament & Brandt, 1998; Parker et al., 2003). Pargament and Brandt (1998) suggest that religious coping is effective because it offers a response to the problems of human insufficiency. When people are pushed beyond the limits of their resources and realize their fundamental vulnerability, religion offers some solutions in the form of spiritual support, explanations for puzzling and difficult life events, and a sense of control. Religion and spirituality can offer interpretations and support that potentially reduce the stress experienced as a result of difficult life circumstances (Pargament & Olsen, 1992). As previously indicated, the beliefs of a religious group can influence the nature of the help given and determine whether the person is viewed as "deserving" of help.

While the support of a relationship with a loving and caring God can be very sustaining for people, depending on circumstances people can also become alienated from or angry with the divine being. Religious responses associated with increased stress include a sense of alienation and dissatisfaction with the religious community, a feeling that God has abandoned one, or a sense of being punished by God (Pargament, 1997; Trenholm, Trent, & Compton, 1998).

A pastor colleague lost his teenage son due to a careless accident on the boy's part. He was very angry with God for letting this tragedy happen. He decided that he finally "had to have it out" with God no matter the cost. After shouting his anger at God, he felt at peace with the silence that for him meant that God understood and accepted his pain and anger. He told his story to a group of community members. One of those present had recently lost his son-in-law in a car accident, leaving his teenage daughter a pregnant widow. He too had been struggling with his anger toward God and was helped in turn to accept and come to terms with his own anger. When he subsequently visited an older woman in the church who had lost her son, he told her of what he had been experiencing. She was then able to share her own feelings of anger and guilt.

Thus the healing of one person became part of a chain of healing for others. The experience of counselors as well as a cursory reading of the headlines of the newspaper or watching the TV news makes it evident that suffering is universal and that people must come to terms with pain and loss in their lives. Suffering is an unavoidable part of the life journey of individuals and families, and understanding how spirituality and the religious context provide meaning during these times can be important in the assessment process.

Rituals

Regardless of their spiritual or religious traditions, rituals often play important roles in the lives of people. Rituals such as graduation from school, entry into marriage, the new beginning of the baseball season, death, and the naming of a child mark life transitions. Rituals play critical roles in spiritual and religious traditions and have deep meaning for those who are part of these traditions. As Streit (2003) indicates, although rituals do not change realities, they help make the meaning of events. Canda and Furman (1999) describe rituals as making and creating transitions, as celebrating them, and as helping us pass through them safely. Inquiring about relevant rituals within spiritual and religious traditions can help identify potential resources for help as well as sources of pain and stress. Social workers can explore with clients the nature of the religious or spiritual rituals that are meaningful to them, the barriers to using these rituals, and the ways clients can draw strengths from the rituals to aid them in healing ways (Van Hook, 2001). Streit (2003) uses the phrase "soul talk" in a moving description of the role of rituals for coping with the pain experienced by individuals, families, and the nation as a result of September 11. "Rituals become powerful vehicles for a person's and a nation's soul to proclaim the full truth of their deepest reactions to horror and sorrow, and the soul's need for hope" (p. 11).

Genograms

Genograms can also be used to incorporate issues related to religion (Frame, 2000; Hodge, 2003a,b). A spiritual genogram can be constructed with the family that specifically addresses the issue of religion, especially as it relates over time to the family story. Social workers can also use the general genogram with clients to incorporate spirituality. Both types of genograms might reveal family estrangements due to an interfaith marriage situation or a change in the belief system or religious affiliation of family members. It might also identify long-term strengths within the family or family messages about religious/spiritual expectations. As a student of the author said long ago, "After doing my family genogram, I realized that I either had to marry a Lutheran pastor or become one." Her choice of marrying a pastor fit with the family's religious prescription. A different life choice might have put her at odds with the family script. Family patterns of religion and spirituality can become disrupted by migrations that place generations in very different cultural/spiritual/religious context from each other. Identifying how spiritual traditions are affected by the migration process (or in turn affect the process) can be a valuable way to understand the impact of the migration experience on individuals and families.

Eco-Maps

Hodge (2003a,b) also describes ways in which the traditional eco-map that identifies the sources of support and strain within the individual or family's current life situation can be used to identify such sources in the area of religion. The church, mosque, temple, synagogue, meeting house, or place of worship, might be a major source of support to one family member while other members might feel alienated from the same resource. Thus expectations from the religious community can be perceived as supports or burdens depending on the particular situation of each family member.

Spiritual Life Maps

Hodge (2003a,b) also describes the technique of spiritual life maps that enable people to tell the story of their journey in a visual manner. Using paper and a variety of drawing supplies or magazines (for pictures), clients can be encouraged to map out their spiritual life. This visual representation then provides the opportunity to discuss these life experiences with the client and enhances understanding of the client's past and present environment and furthers the healing process.

LIFE CYCLE ISSUES

Childhood

Children are typically introduced to religious traditions through their parents and other close family members. Images of divinity are not only created by what parents teach their children, but also are personified by the nature of relationships within the family. For example, if a childhood experience of parents is judgmental, distant, and/or critical, such experiences may be reflected in the individual's images of God. "God the father" thus becomes yet another powerful figure who is likely to be judgmental and rejecting of the individual. On the other hand, loving relationships within the family can help children establish trusting relationships with the transcendent. These early experiences often form the basis for later religious and spiritual journeys.

Adolescence

Adolescence is a time for establishing personal identities in the area of spirituality and religion as well as in other areas of life. For some young people, this can be a time of questioning the beliefs of the family and creating their own spiritual/religious beliefs, practices, and interpersonal ties.

Adults

Religious traditions frequently have important prescriptions regarding adult relationships within the context of marriage and parenthood. Spiritual aspects of life related to meaning can become important as people establish these central relationships and take on the responsibility of parenthood. This is also typically the time during which individuals forge their own religious or spiritual identities. Because this is influenced by a myriad of life events, the individual's religious or spiritual identity may change throughout the life cycle.

Older adults can have a wide range of spiritual needs that include: the need for meaning, purpose, and hope; the need to transcend circumstances; a need for support in dealing with loss; a need for continuity; a need for validation and support of their religious behavior; a need to engage in religious behaviors; a need for personal dignity and a sense of worthiness; a need for unconditional love; a need to express anger and doubt; a need to feel that God is on their side; a need to love and serve others; a need to be thankful; a need to forgive and be forgiven; and a need to prepare for death and dying (Watkins, 2001).

Aging

Aging is a time of loss—of friends and family members, of social roles, of physical abilities. These changes have spiritual implications that can be experienced as depressing or as opportunities for spiritual growth and development (Moberg, 2001a).

Important spiritual needs frequently emerge as people enter the later stages of life: the need for meaning and purpose, the need for love and relatedness, the need for forgiveness, and the need for spiritual integration (Moberg, 2001d). As people review their lives and cope with the problems facing them now, there is a need for a sense of meaning for the specific events of daily life and for the ultimate meaning of life. This need for meaning is related to the wish to maintain a sense of dignity and self-esteem (Moberg, 2001d). People need a sense of being loved as they are. Religion for some people offers this sense of being loved in this way. The need for forgiveness is also important because people tend to carry with them shame or guilt for what they have done wrong or failed to have done or have unresolved guilt (Moberg, 2001d). A recent study of older adults living in the community found that seeking forgiveness was one of the major coping strategies identified by respondents, especially by women (Van Hook & Rivera, 2004). There is also a need to maintain ourselves in a spiritual manner beyond our biological existence. For some people this is reflected in hope for immortality of some type (Moberg, 2001d).

Difficult times during the life cycle can evoke anger toward God with an accompanying sense of guilt for this anger. A listening and understanding stance is important during these times. Use of metaphors of God as a parent who understands hurt and anger just as human parents do can be helpful if appropriate for the religious context of the person.

TREATMENT APPROACHES

Incorporating spirituality and related religion in the counseling process can take a variety of forms and is dependent on the nature of the problem and the tradition of the person. Two important questions can help identify potential resources. How have people accessed resources from their spiritual/religious frameworks in the past to address problems? What resources might be present that are not being used that could be marshaled to deal with the current life events?

It is important to engage clients in a dialogue to identify what resources might be present within their spiritual life or religious tradition. Such an approach respects the expert role of clients in contributing their knowledge to the healing process. Counselors can thus be partners with clients in the identification of what ways constitute healing and what ways exist to facilitate this part of the life journey. Previously described directed therapeutic conversations and assessment techniques can help the process of dialogue. The following discussion describes some specific approaches that incorporate spirituality/religion, such as a relationship with the divine-being, rituals, meditation, journaling, and participation in the religious community. The specific meaning and content of these will vary widely depending on the nature of the problem, the person, and the traditions.

Hodge (2003b) describes several empirically based spiritual resources that may be used in a treatment model that incorporates spirituality/religion. The relationship with the Ultimate (as identified within various traditions) is a key resource that facilitates coping, defeats loneliness, promotes a sense of purpose in life, helps one gain a sense of personal worth and value, and provides hope for the future. Rituals that are part of every spiritual tradition have been associated with positive outcomes in terms of easing anxiety, reducing isolation, promoting feelings of security, and feeling loved and cared for. Participation in a religious community (through religious services, membership in groups, celebrations) has also given people both a sense of belonging and of strength. A belief system that gives one a sense of being loved and having a purpose in life also supports resiliency. Hodge reminds us that ultimately it is the client's own interpretation that determines the impact of these aspects of spirituality and religion on his or her life.

Meditation

Meditation plays an important role in many different spiritual/ religious traditions. This topic is addressed in depth in Chapter 2, "Mindfulness, Meditation, and Health," and thus is not addressed here.

Rituals

Rituals from spiritual/religious traditions can be powerful instruments for healing. The following section includes some of the religious rituals among selected religious traditions and demonstrates the widespread nature of these rituals. The vast number of religious traditions and rituals within these traditions precludes a complete discussion.

Brave Heart (2001) describes the role of one of the sacred rites of the Lakota, *hunka,* which is the "making of relatives" ceremony. This rite is "a traditional adoption ceremony that binds the participants' spirits, creating a relationship that is considered more sacred than biological kinship" (Brave Heart, p. 22). Such a ceremony enables people to extend their *tiospaye* (collection of related families) and create surrogate families when biological families have been lost due to death or when people are estranged from their biological family. The Sweat Lodge ceremony plays an important role as a means of purification in most of the Native Peoples' nations.

Hinduism has developed a variety of rituals in which the entire family participates. The aim of these rituals is to strengthen the family bond and to fulfill "social dharma—one's duties and responsibilities to the family, community, and the world at large" (Singh, 2001, p. 43). These rituals prepare people for the cyclical stages of life from birth to death. Buddhism has many rituals for family and religious community events. Although specific rituals vary depending on the particular sect, all types of Buddhism encourage meditation to calm and clear the mind as a basis for all other spiritual practices (Canda, 2001). Confucianism supports respect of the ancestors through important rituals that honor the dead as well as other life cycle rituals that recognize the importance of the family and education (Chung, 2001). The Jewish tradition has a calendar marked by a series of celebrations and holy days with their accompanying set of rituals. These events memorialize the past and its lessons for the present and the identity of the Jewish people (Friedman, 2001). Even Jewish people who do not go to the synagogue on a regular basis join family members to celebrate these important holy days and celebrations. Within the Islamic faith, important rituals are included as part of the obligatory duties for Muslims. These include the Declaration of Faith (the *shahadah*), the five daily prayers, the fast of Ramadan, and the pilgrimage to Makkah (the *Hajii*) (Nadir & Dziegielewski, 2001).

The Catholic tradition has sacraments that mark important life cycle milestones from birth to death and maintain the connection between human beings and God. Both Catholic sacraments and other rituals are further influenced by the unique ethnic backgrounds of participants. These celebrations represent "memory stones" that "mark the particular place, moment in time or part of human life made sacred by the meeting of the mystery of God with the mystery of the human creation." (Aguilar, 2001, p. 126). Protestant Christian groups differ somewhat in the nature of their specific rituals but both individual and group prayers are important for all denominations. Communion (or the Lord's Supper) is an important ritual within Protestant, Catholic, and Orthodox traditions through which participants remember the death of Christ as a sacrifice for them. Seventh-Day Adventists practice the ritual of foot washing prior to Communion as a way of making amends to others and as a symbolic act of humility (Vander Waal & McMullim, 2001). Baptism in various forms is an important symbol of membership in the family of God (Scales, 2001; Van Hook, 2001). Mormons conduct the ritual of baptism of the dead within their temples (Haynes, 2001). A church service within the African-American tradition may be full of emotional connection with God and one's fellow worshippers through music and the pattern of call and response between pastor and congregation (Grant, 2001).

For individuals whose spirituality is part of identifying with a religious tradition, the rituals associated with their tradition can be powerful aids in the healing process. Inability to participate in rituals due to physical frailty, geographic distance, or sense of alienation can cause distress. Failure to carry out important rituals can create tension within families while exclusion by other family members from important rituals can create lasting hurt.

A medical social worker shared the following example of the power of drawing on the customs of culture and spirituality.

An older hospitalized woman was suffering from great pain. When she refused pain medication, the social worker was urged by the medical staff to institute the process of involuntary commitment. The social worker, sensitive to possible cultural and spiritual resources within the life space of the client, engaged the family as allies. The extended family came, formed a circle around the patient, and began to sing music from their traditional religion. The effect on the woman was remarkable. The sounds of the music and the healing touch of her family helped the pain to recede. She had come from a poor Caribbean community in which access to medication was very limited and in which people developed rituals for healing that evoked music and the spiritual power of the community to address issues of pain and illness.

Clients and counselors together can also create rituals that are meaningful for the client and the setting. Such rituals may involve the religious or cultural background of the client or can be created as a unique response to a situation. Everyday items can become powerful symbols to enhance these rituals. Streit (2003) describes how a piece of clothing used by a lost loved one can become an important symbol and play a critical role in the ritual. Such an item can be used as a token of memory or can in some other way evoke the special presence of the loved one. Canda and Furman (1999) describe the process of working with clients to create personal rituals. They organize this process in 10 steps:

(1) Identify your intention,
(2) Symbolize your purpose and hope,
(3) Symbolize the process of celebration or change (what actions will occur),
(4) Create a meaningful time and place,
(5) Invite supportive participants (or meaningful nonhuman beings),
(6) Open the ritual or ceremony,
(7) Enact the celebration or transformation,
(8) Make a commitment to the future,
(9) Give gratitude, and
(10) Close the ritual or ceremony. (p. 305)

The design of the ritual represents a thoughtful process and the actual process of designing the ritual plays a part in the healing process.

Social Support

Social support from the religious or spiritual communities may represent important resources and social workers can be instrumental in connecting people with members of the religious or spiritual community. These ties can be with religious leaders or other members of the community. In addressing sensitive religious matters, leaders from the religious community can potentially bring healing messages and approaches that can be very powerful.

As a social work student the author began working with a Catholic woman whose child had recently been born blind. She was very depressed, not only by the child's disability, but also because she interpreted it as punishment from God. In the context of pre-Vatican II, she had previously been divorced and had subsequently remarried. Since her divorce was contrary to church teaching, she had not participated in confession (the sacrament of reconciliation) or mass since that time. She had been waiting for God to punish her for this. When her baby was born blind, she was sure that it was God's punishment and that she was guilty for her child's condition. Fortunately, the author's supervisor was knowledgeable about resources within the Catholic Church in New York City. We contacted a group of Roman Catholic nuns who visited her and assured her that this was not a punishment from God. She was encouraged to meet with a supportive priest. These interventions by members of the religious community were powerful in releasing her from the painful burden of guilt and enabled her to cope with the child's condition.

Some religious congregations have professionally trained counselors or lay volunteers who are trained and willing to be supportive partners with others for a variety of needs. The Stephens ministry within many Protestant groups, The Ministry to the Sick and a long list of other programs within The Catholic Church, and the Social Service Department within the Islamic tradition (organized either through the local mosque of the community Islamic society) are examples of resources available to clients. These programs train and support members to be of help to others of all ages and can be invaluable resources to individuals and families during difficult times. Many religious communities also have resources that are organized either directly by the congregation or through organizations supported by the faith community to provide clients with food, clothing, and other material needs. Such programs reflect the central concern of caring for members of the church and the community that is at the core of their religious faith and tradition.

Life Review

Life review can be a way to help people identify and address some of their spiritual needs. While the life review is frequently described as a resource for older adults, it can also be used throughout the life span (Moberg, 2001d). Incorporating spiritual issues within the life review can be a valuable experience, especially when shared with a sympathetic audience. In order to facilitate the healing process, such a life review should include the dark valleys of pain and doubt as well as the peaks of joy and peace (Moberg, 2001d). During the process of life review, a person is helped to create a sense of meaning of her or his life and to recognize how individual events fit into the context of life as a whole. "Life review therapy helps to reintegrate unresolved conflicts, and fears, expiate guilt feelings, reconcile broken family relationships, and prepare the person for a peaceful death" (Moberg,

2001d, p. 160). Clients can be helped to recognize their contributions to those around them during their life. As Chaplain Ison (1998) has written, "Telling the story of one's life is like weaving a tapestry with symbolic ribbons of family, faith, health, hope, joy, death, love, adversity, and much more, that creates 'a weaving of great beauty, significance and holiness'" (p. 3). Counselors must be aware that sometimes a life review can result in despair and extreme feelings of regret. These responses are sometimes prompted by unrealistic expectations and a cultural context that values youth. The counselor needs to help individuals also recognize the positive aspects of their lives. The ability to be useful to others is an important human need that promotes self-respect. Counselors can help people identify ways that they can still contribute despite poor health and limited economic resources through offering encouraging words or a listening ear that support the spiritual life of others (Koenig, 1999).

Spiritual Legacy

The spiritual legacy revolves around the issue of "for what do I want to be remembered spiritually?" After one has answered this question, Moberg (2001b) raises three additional questions: "(1) What have I already done that contributed to that objective? (2) What am I doing and being now to bring that memory to others? and (3) What can I do during the rest of my life to make more certain that I will attain that goal?" (p. 172). This approach is grounded in the ancient Jewish traditions included in "Hebrew Ethical Will" by which fathers conveyed ethical guidelines to their children and encouraged them to remain faithful to the Jewish tradition. Cohen (2004) describes a contemporary version built on the concept of the life review described earlier. Components of this spiritual legacy include: a resiliency focus, reflection of who one is, what one has learned from important milestones and events in life, who have been important people in one's life, the important values and beliefs in one's life, and the values, beliefs, and lessons that one wishes to leave one's family and friends. While these spiritual legacies have been associated with older adults, Cohen indicates that they can also be valuable during other important times of life, for example, marriage, birth of a child, baptism, bar/bat mitzvah, divorce, or surgery.

Journaling

Journaling is an effective tool generally in the counseling process that can also be used to discover and explore spiritual aspects of life. Counselors can encourage people to look at meaning of life issues in their journaling process (Canda & Furman, 1999; Frame, 2003). Journaling can also play a valuable role in clarifying one's own values and beliefs for counseling as part of the important self-reflection process (Canda & Furman, 1999).

Visualization

Visualization and related spiritual imagery represent another technique that can be used to address issues. People are asked to close their eyes and imagine scenes. They can then be led on a narrative journey to help them identify meaningful issues (Frame, 2003).

Literature and Art

Literature and the visual arts can be important spiritual resources. People can be encouraged to read literature or explore the art forms in the spiritual traditions that are appropriate for them (Canda & Furman, 1999) or have meaning for them. The key issue here is to work with clients to identify literature and art within their traditions to avoid the trap of counselors imposing their own views on clients. Frame (2003) cites the need to choose these pieces carefully lest one select pieces that are overly simplistic, which leads to failure in recognizing the complexities of life, or pieces that are too complicated, as they include so many problems that people can feel overwhelmed.

Forgiveness

Forgiveness of self and others is also a powerful therapeutic process and has been associated with improved mental and physical health (Canda & Furman, 1999; Frame, 2003). While forgiveness is supported by many religious traditions, the meaning of forgiveness varies depending on the tradition. As a result, counselors need to seek understanding about the meaning of forgiveness within the client's tradition. The God of Christianity, Judaism, and Islam models forgiveness. In Judaism only the injured can grant forgiveness. Within Eastern religious traditions, harmful actions are viewed within a concept of worldwide suffering. Offenses are viewed as resulting more from ignorance than evil so that forgiveness arises out of compassion for others (Frame, 2003, p. 195).

It is important to delineate between forgiveness and reconciliation. The latter implies that the offending party has apologized for what he or she has done and that a relationship between the two parties is restored. Reconciliation thus requires actions on the part of both the offender and the person who has been hurt. Forgiveness, on the other hand, can occur even when the other party is not aware of this process. Thus forgiveness and its possible healing are not held hostage to the actions of the offending party. Freedman (1998), as cited in Frame (2003), describes four options that can be discussed with clients in this regard: "(1) forgive and reconcile, (2) forgive and not reconcile, (3) not forgive and interact, (4) not forgive and not reconcile" (p. 195). While people can be educated about the price one has to pay for living without forgiving, such a decision is naturally that of the client and further exploration of issues may well be needed. Forgiveness is also not forgetting. While one can let go of the anger, it may still be important to recognize the danger in the situation and to exercise self-protection. A spouse who has experienced domestic violence and left the scene of the abuse may in time be able to forgive the abusing partner. At the same time, if the partner has not changed, it is crucial that she remember the danger and avoid placing herself at risk again.

Frame (2003) describes the stages identified by Richards and Bergin (1997) when people are ready to move toward forgiveness. These stages include:

(1) shock and denial,
(2) awareness of the hurt or abuse,
(3) acknowledgement of the grief, and anger, and the opportunity to express their feelings to others,
(4) validation of their feelings,
(5) justice and restitution if possible,
(6) prevention of further offences, and
(7) forgiveness and moving on. (p. 195)

Forgiving oneself may be as difficult as forgiving others. Counselors may need to help people develop empathy for themselves and find ways to accept grace or perhaps to make appropriate amends to the person who was injured. Making amends may be complicated when the injured party is no longer living or available. Sometimes people can make amends to another person.

Bill was the son of a leading member of a small religiously conservative community. While in high school he made his girlfriend pregnant and felt that he had disgraced his father. He left town and spent the years that followed trying to run away from his sense of shame and guilt. He tried drugs, the military, and then drugs again. The further he ran away, the heavier he felt his burden of guilt. Finally with treatment he was able to overcome his drug addiction and return to his home community. Bill's father, however, had died suddenly before he returned so that he could not ask for his father's forgiveness and seek restitution in this manner. The counselor arranged for a meeting between Bill and his mother. He was able to explain to his mother how much he loved his father and how he felt that he had let the family down, especially his father. He explained that he has been running away because of these feelings. His mother's interpretation during these years had been that Bill did not care about his father. The reconciliation between Bill and his mother was based on her new understanding of the clear sorrow of Bill and provided a powerful basis for healing within both Bill and his mother. Through his mother Bill also felt reconciled with his father.

Rituals can be valuable in terms of forgiveness. People can write a note to the offending party and then read it to the counselor or other trusted parties. Letters of anger or apology have been read to the tombstone of people who have died. Candles can be lighted to signify the new life.

While forgiveness can be healing, counselors need to be aware of pressure on people to forgive and therefore need to allow them to make their own choices in this regard. Sometimes people within the religious community or the family circle pressure people to forgive, hoping that this will end a problem situation and bring some magical sense of closure. Counselors need to affirm the right of people to make their own choices and to recognize that a process is involved. As indicated in the following example, sometimes this means supporting people in the process of protecting themselves and their family members and in countering pressure from others.

A family was referred to the author by a pastor because their daughter refused to forgive her grandfather who had sexually abused her. When pressured by a previous counselor and her pastor to forgive the grandfather who had sexually abused many members of the family, everyone else in the family circle stated that they would forgive. An older sister said the required words that she would forgive him but also stated that she refused to ever see him again. The circle stopped when the client refused to forgive. The grandfather had never said that he was sorry for what he had done and had not listened to the words of hurt by the girls. The author indicated to the pastor that forgiveness was a process and that he would work with the family but not with the expectation that the client had to forgive her grandfather. In this situation the parents needed to be strengthened in their role and their right to protect their daughters and to make whatever decisions supported their family. Some months later, the grandparents and parents met with their respective counselors. During this meeting the grandfather finally said that he realized he had hurt his granddaughters, was sorry for what he had done, and asked for forgiveness. The parents indicated that they would convey these words to their girls but also set very clear ground rules for any contacts between the children and the grandparents.

CONCLUSION

Spirituality can be an important resource for some individuals to promote healing. Opening the door to this resource requires self-reflection on the part of the counselor, respect for the role of spirituality and/or religion in the lives of others, and a willingness to work with clients in a truly collaborative manner. Clients need to be assured that counselors value this aspect of their life.

This chapter began with a list of activities that might be reflections of spirituality. This list is naturally only a small sample of activities that can be supportive of spirituality. Including spirituality within the counseling process requires knowledge of possibilities, but even more so openness to exploring the meaningful activities for the individuals involved. While walking a labyrinth might be deeply meaningful to one person, for another a walk in the woods, listening to music, or reading spiritual literature might be a much more powerful spiritual experience. Lighting a candle, journaling, praying, sharing one's dreams with a friend, or participating in a traditional religious ritual all represent only possibilities. Drawing on spirituality in the counseling process brings us back to the collaborative healing relationship. Such a relationship provides the context for conveying caring, exploring important issues of meaning, and identifying activities that enhance spiritual resources that can promote the healing process.

REFERENCES

Aguilar, M. (2001). Catholicism. In M. Van Hook, B. Hugen, & M. Aguilar (Eds.), *Spirituality within religious traditions in social work practice* (pp. 120-145). Pacific Grove: Brooks Cole.

ben Asher, M. (2001). Spirituality and religion social work practice. *Social Work Today, 1*(7), 14-18.

Booth, J. & Martin, J.E. (1998). Spiritual and religious factors in substance use, dependence and recover. In H. Koenig (Ed.), *Handbook of religion and mental health* (pp. 175-199). New York: Academic Press.

Brave Heart, M.Y. (2001). Lakota—Native people's spirituality. In M. Van Hook, B. Hugen, & M. Aguilar (Eds.), *Spirituality within religious traditions in social work practice* (pp. 18-33). Pacific Grove: Brooks Cole.

Bullis, R. (1996). *Spirituality in social work practice.* Washington, DC: Taylor & Francis.

Canda, E. (1997). Does religion and spirituality have a significant place in the core HBSE curriculum? Yes. In M. Bloom & W.C. Klein (Eds.), *Controversial issues in human behavior and the social environment* (pp. 172-177). Boston: Allyn & Bacon.

Canda, E. (2001). Buddhism. In M. Van Hook, B. Hugen, & M. Aguilar (Eds.), *Spirituality within religious traditions in social work practice* (pp. 53-72). Pacific Grove: Brooks Cole.

Canda, E.R. & Furman, L.D. (1999). *Spiritual diversity in social work practice.* New York: Free Press.

Cascio, T. (1998). Incorporating spirituality into social work practice: A review of what to do. *Families in Society: The Journal of Contemporary Human Services, 79*(5), 523-531.

Chung, D. (2001). Confucianism. In M. Van Hook, B. Hugen, & M. Aguilar (Eds.), *Spirituality within religious traditions in social work practice* (pp. 73-97). Pacific Grove: Brooks Cole.

Cohen, H.L. (2004, February). *Creating a spiritual legacy.* Paper presented at the Second National Gerontological Social Work Conference in Conjunction with the Council on Social Work Education, Anaheim, CA.

Cummings, S., Neff, J., & Husaini, B. (2003). Functional impairments as a predictor of depressive symptomatology: The role of race, religiosity, and social support. *Health and Social Work, 28*(1), 23-32.

Donahue, M.J. & Benson, P.L. (1995). Religion and the well-being of adolescents. *Journal of Social Issues, 51*(2), 145-160.

Dossey, B. & Dossey, M. (1998). Body-mind spirit: Attending to holistic care. *American Journal of Nursing, 98*(8), 35-38.

Folwarski, J. & Marganoff, P. (1996). Polish families. In M. McGolderick, J. Giordano, & J. Pearce (Eds.), *Ethnicity and family therapy* (2nd ed.) (pp. 658-672). New York: Guilford Press.

Frame, M.W. (2000). The spiritual genogram in family therapy. *Journal of Marital and Family Therapy, 26*(2), 211-216.

Frame, M.W. (2003). *Integrating religion and spirituality into counseling: A comprehensive approach.* Pacific Grove: Brooks Cole.

Freedman, S. (1998). Forgiveness and reconciliation: The importance of understanding how they differ. *Counseling and Values, 42,* 100-116 as cited in Frame, M.W. (2003). *Integrating religion and spirituality into counseling: A comprehensive approach.* Pacific Grove: Brooks Cole.

Friedman, B. (2001). Judaism. In M. Van Hook, B. Hugen, & M. Aguilar (Eds.), *Spirituality within religious traditions in social work practice* (pp. 98-119). Pacific Grove: Brooks Cole.

Garcia-Preto, N. (1996). Puerto-Rican families. In M. McGolderick, J. Giordano, & J. Pearce. (Eds.), *Ethnicity and family therapy* (2nd ed.) (pp. 183-199). New York: The Guilford Press.

Gibson, M. (Producer/Director). (2004). *The passion of the Christ.* Icon Productions.

Giordano, J. & McGolderick, M. (1996). Italian families. In M. McGolderick, J. Giordano, & J. Pearce (Eds.), *Ethnicity and family therapy* (pp. 567-582). New York: Guilford Press.

Gordon, E.W. & Song, L.D. (1994). Variations in the experience of resilience. In M.C. Wang & E.W. Gordon (Eds.), *Educational resilience in inner-city America: Challenges and prospects* (pp. 27-43). Hillsdale, NJ: Lawrence Erlbaum.

Grant, D. (2001). The African American Baptist tradition. In M. Van Hook, B. Hugen, & M. Aguilar (Eds.), *Spirituality within religious traditions in social work practice* (pp. 205-227). Pacific Grove: Brooks Cole.

Haynes, D. (2001). Mormonism. In M. Van Hook, B. Hugen, & M. Aguilar (Eds.), *Spirituality within religious traditions in social work practice* (pp. 251-272). Pacific Grove: Brooks Cole.

Hodge, D.R. (2003a). Assessing client spirituality: Understanding the advantages of utilizing different assessment approaches. *Society for Spirituality and Social Work Forum, 10*(1), 8-10.

Hodge, D.R. (2003b). *Spiritual assessment: Handbook for helping professionals.* Botsford, CT. North American Association of Christian Social Workers.

Hugen, B. (2001). Spirituality and religion in social work practice: A conceptual model. In M. Van Hook, B. Hugen, & M. Aguilar (Eds.), *Spirituality within religious traditions and social work practice* (pp. 9-17). Pacific Grove: Brooks Cole.

Ison, C. (1998). A tapestry of life. *Aging and Religion, 2,* 1-8.

Jacobs, C. (1997). Essay on spirituality and social work practice. *Smith College Studies in Social Work, 67*(2), 171-175.

Koenig, E. (1994). *Aging and God: Spiritual pathways to mental health in midlife and later years.* Binghamton, NY: The Haworth Press.

Koenig, H. (1999). *The healing power of faith: Science explores medicine's last great frontier.* New York: Simon and Schuster.

Koenig, H. (2000). Religion, well-being and health in the elderly: The scientific evidence for an association. In J. Thorson (Ed.), *Perspectives in spiritual well-being and aging* (pp. 84-97). Springfield, IL: C.T. Thomas.

Koenig, H.G., George, L.K., & Titus, P. (2004). Religion, spirituality, and health in medically ill hospitalized older patients. *Journal of American Geriatric Society, 52*(4), 554-562.

Levin, J.S. & Chatters, L. (1998). Research on religion and mental health: An overview of empirical findings and theoretical issues. In H. Koenig (Ed.), *Handbook of religion and mental health issues* (pp. 33-50). New York: Academic Press.

McGolderick, M. (1996). Irish families. In M. McGolderick, J. Giordano, & J. Pearce (Eds.), *Ethnicity and family therapy* (2nd ed.) (pp. 544-566). New York: Guilford Press.

Moberg, D. (2001a). *Aging and spirituality: Spiritual dimensions of aging theory, research, and policy.* Binghamton, NY: Haworth Press.

Moberg, D. (2001b). The reality and centrality of spirituality. In D. Moberg (Ed.), *Aging and spirituality: Spiritual dimensions of aging theory, research, and policy* (pp. 3-20). Binghamton, NY: Haworth Press.

Moberg, D. (2001c). Research on spirituality. In D. Moberg (Ed.), *Aging and spirituality: Spiritual dimensions of aging theory, research, and policy* (pp. 55-70). Binghamton, NY: Haworth Press.

Moberg, D. (2001d). The spiritual life review. In D. Moberg (Ed.), *Aging and spirituality: Spiritual dimensions of aging theory, research, and policy* (pp. 159-176). Binghamton, NY: Haworth Press.

Nadir, A. & Dziegielewski, S. (2001). Islam. In M. VanHook, B. Hugen, & M. Aguilar (Eds.), *Spirituality within religious traditions and social work practice* (pp. 146-166). Pacific Grove: Brooks Cole.

Pargament, K. (1997). *The psychology of religion and coping: Theory, research, and practice.* New York: The Guilford Press.

Pargament, K.I. & Brandt, C.R. (1998). Religion in coping. In H. Koenig (Ed.), *Handbook of religion and mental health* (pp. 111-128). New York: Academic Press.

Pargament, K.I. & Olsen, H. (1992). God help me (II): The relationship of religious orientations to religious coping with negative life events. *Journal of the Scientific Study of Religion, 31*(4), 504-513.

Parker, M., Roff, L., Klemmack, D., Koenig, H., Baker, P., & Allman, R. (2003). Religiosity and mental health in southern, community-dwelling older adults. *Aging and Mental Health, 7*(5), 390-397.

Perry, B.G. (1998). The relationship between faith and well-being. *Journal of Religion and Health, 37*(2), 125.

Richards, P.S. & Bergin, A.E. (1997). *A spiritual strategy for counseling and psychotherapy.* Washington, DC: American Psychological Association.

Roff, L., Klemmack, D., Parker, M., Koenig, H., Crowther, M., Baker, P., & Allman, R. (2004). *Depression and religiosity in African American and white community-dwelling older adults.*

Scales, T.L. (2001). Baptists. In M. VanHook, B. Hugen, & M. Aguilar (Eds.), *Spirituality within religious traditions and social work practice* (pp. 185-204). Pacific Grove: Brooks Cole.

Seeleby, D.D. (1992). *The strengths perspective in social work practice.* New York: Longman.

Sherwood, D. (2002). Ethical integration of faith and social work practice: Evangelism. *Social Work and Christianity, 29*(1), 1-12.

Singh, R. (2001). Hinduism. In M. Van Hook, B. Hugen, & M. Aguilar (Eds.), *Spirituality within religious traditions in social work practice* (pp. 9-17). Pacific Grove: Brooks Cole.

Streit, D. (2003). Rituals say it with feeling. *Society for Spirituality and Social Work Forum, 10*(1), 11-13.

Thayne, T. (1998). Opening space for client's religious spiritual values in therapy: A social constructionist perspective. *Journal of Family Social Work, 2*(4), 13-23.

Trenholm, P., Trent J., & Compton, A. (1998). Negative religious conflict as a predictor of panic disorder. *Journal of Clinical Psychology, 54*(1), 59-65.

Van Hook, M. (2001). Protestantism. In M. Van Hook, B. Hugen, & M. Aguilar (Eds.), *Spirituality within religious traditions in social work practice* (pp. 267-183). Pacific Grove: Brooks Cole.

Van Hook, M. & Aguilar, M. (2001). Health, religion, and spirituality. In M. Van Hook, B. Hugen, & M. Aguilar (Eds.), *Spirituality within religious traditions in social work practice* (pp. 273-289). Pacific Grove: Brooks Cole.

Van Hook, M., Hugen, B., & Aguilar, M. (2001). *Spirituality within religious traditions in social work practice.* Pacific Grove: Brooks Cole.

Van Hook, M. & Rivera, J.O. (in press). *Coping with difficult life transitions by older adults: The role of religion.*

Vander Waal, C. & McMullen, D. (2001). Seventh-Day Adventists. In M. Van Hook, B. Hugen, & M. Aguilar (Eds.), *Spirituality within religious traditions in social work practice* (pp. 228-250). Pacific Grove: Brooks Cole.

Walsh, F. (1998). *Strengthening family resilience.* New York: The Guilford Press.

Walsh, F. (1999). Opening family therapy to spirituality. In F. Walsh (Ed.), *Spiritual resources in family therapy* (pp. 28-60). New York: The Guilford Press.

Walsh, F. (1999). Religion and spirituality: Wellsprings for healing and resilience. In F. Walsh, (Ed.), *Spiritual resources in family therapy* (pp. 3-27). New York: The Guilford Press.

Walsh, F. (1999). *Spiritual resources in family therapy.* New York: The Guilford Press.

Watkins, D. (2001). Spirituality in social work practice with older persons. In D. Moberg (Ed.), *Aging and spirituality: Spiritual dimensions of aging theory, research, practice, and policy* (pp. 133-146). Binghamton, NY: Haworth Press.

Werner, E.E. & Smith, R. (1992). *Overcoming the odds: High risk children from birth to adulthood.* Ithaca, NY: Cornell University Press.

White, M. & Epston, D. (1990). *Narrative means to therapeutic ends.* New York: Norton.

Wright, L. (1999). Spirituality, suffering, and beliefs: The soul of healing with families. In F. Walsh (Ed.), *Spiritual resources in family therapy* (pp. 61-75). New York: The Guilford Press.

Chapter 4

Tearing the Darkness Down: Poetry As Therapy

Perie J. Longo

I didn't trust it for a moment
but I drank it anyway,
the wine of my own poetry.

It gave me the daring to take hold
of the darkness and tear it down
and cut it into little pieces.

Lalla, Fourteenth century,
Persian (Barks, 1992)

INTRODUCTION

From the time we are conceived in our mother's womb, we are born to the rhythm of the heart, the movement of step. We grow in the fluid darkness taking nourishment from the placenta, stretching and kicking until one day we work our way into light, a fully formed human being ready to take on life. Already the makings of poetry are part of our nature. With our first cry we make our first poem, with one breath and the next, a sound that reverberates in our mother's heart and when she cries in response, we hear our first poem. And so it continues, the voices of those who care for us convey all the emotions we will come to know as our own, words that if written down would be

Introduction to Alternative and Complementary Therapies
© 2008 by The Haworth Press, Taylor & Francis Group. All rights reserved.
doi:10.1300/5987_04

poetry. It is that simple. Poetry is giving sound and rhythm to silence, to darkness, giving it a shape, turning it to light. When we read a poem that can be related with our experiences, there is a shift, a click within. Someone has understood our darkness by naming their own. We feel less alone. When we harness emotion to the page, we understand ourselves better, and eventually others. Therapeutically, the "I" gathers energy and insight. Our world expands (Longo, 2006).

When I was very young, my father would make me sit on his lap before bedtime, bounce me on his knee, and recite Longfellow's "Listen my child and you shall hear/Of the midnight ride of Paul Revere." I can still feel the rhythms burrowing into my body. I would take this pleasure into sleep, no longer afraid of the darkness, and listen to my thoughts. Later on, in early elementary school days, when I would get bored in school, I would start moving my feet to some rhythm and words would flow automatically. Though I didn't write them down, I would feel comforted and be able to return to the moment. It is poetry's nature to comfort and sustain through rhythm, which has the power to unlock emotion. Poetry has been my friend, guide, and fortification ever since. Through writing poetry, I have come to know myself. I have learned to voice my thoughts.

Only a few hours after the tragedy of 9/11, I heard Billy Collins, poet laureate at the time, interviewed on NPR. As I drove my car to work in a fog, the billowing smoke I saw on television still lingering in my vision and feeling numb, I heard the interviewer say that it is during times of tragedy we turn to poetry. Was there one he would recommend? Collins replied he would read Mary Oliver's "Wild Geese" which contains the line "Tell me about despair, yours, and I will tell you mine" (Oliver, 1993). With these words I took a deep breath, relieved that what we all felt was being honored. We would speak our despair and speak our stories in an attempt to assuage our shock and loss, to try and understand, make sense of the impossible, to look for the meaning in such horror. We would try to find words for the mystery. That is what has drawn many of us to the field of poetry therapy.

Poetry therapy, bibliotherapy, and journal therapy, terms used synonymously, are contemporary terms for practices that have evolved through time. The National Association for Poetry Therapy (NAPT) describes writing for healing as "the intentional use of the written or spoken word by a trained biblio/poetry/journal therapist to further therapeutic goals and enhance the well-being of individuals and groups through the integration of emotional, cognitive, and social aspects of self" (NAPT, circa 1996). Many of us working in the field stumbled across poetry therapy while doing a research paper for school. Perhaps we loved poetry because we were English majors or maybe we read a poem that spoke to us and lifted our heart out of some darkness. Perhaps we came across the book *Poetry Therapy* by Jack J. Leedy (1969), "the father of poetry therapy," which is how I became involved.

I had been working for a year through California-poets-in-the-schools and was so impressed with the therapeutic benefit of children's written response to hearing good poetry, that I returned to school to get my degree in psychology. I wanted to know how poetry helped children shine. Each week when I came to teach a class, they would applaud and yell "Poetry Time." One child wrote, "Poetry is better than Disneyland." Often I would observe the shyest child transform until she or he couldn't wait to read a personal poem. Children often wrote that poetry "makes me feel better about myself." Teachers often commented to me how children who often had the most difficulty with language in school are the ones who gain the most from the poetry classes.

LANGUAGE AND POETRY

In the Inuit language, the root word *anerca* means both to breathe and to make poetry: an inseparable act. The Navajos have a similar notion. The in-breath is the First Holy One, Thought or Long Life; the out-breath is the Second Holy One, and when articulated, is speech and beauty. Language in its perfection is the chant, is the poem that has a powerful impact on our lives and the ability to heal and that which shapes our world (Witherspoon, 1977). Language from a primitive stance is sacred, is life itself. For many, poetry is food for the soul and carries them to deeply meaningful places. Often I have heard people say "poetry saved my life." Jack J. Leedy (1985) has said,

> Poetry is the royal road to the unconscious and a natural healing vehicle to encouraging communication . . . a secret power and an untapped national resource for healing. Poetry is a guide to the hidden mind and to a more creative and enriching life. (p. xxii)

However, when the two words "poetry" and "therapy" are uttered together, there is an unpleasant reaction at times. This is peculiar since language is our primary mode of communication. Standing in line after a psychology workshop one afternoon, to collect our continuing education certificates, a colleague turned to me and asked, "Are you still doing poetry therapy?" When I said I was, she said, "I hate poetry," and turned away. At first I was taken aback, but later thought she was most likely uncomfortable with how poets use language, or that she had not read much contemporary poetry. The self-expressive creative arts of art, dance, music, and drama seem more accessible and popular than poetry, which seems to be the "slowest creative art to gain recognition for the healing and growth potential it possesses" (Kemplar, 2003, p. 218). This may be in part due to the popularization of the other arts in schools and in marketing.

Poetry also has long been engulfed in a shadow of mysticism, perhaps because it seems too remote, the language removed from daily conversation. The main character of poetry, after all, is language where poets find great pleasure in maneuvering sounds and words to capture a moment or a mood. They experiment to find new ways to say the familiar so that we will pay attention to or cast a new light on things that would otherwise be ignored.

Once, when I suggested to a novelist to write a poem about something that moved him, he said, "I don't have time. It would take years for me to write a poem, and besides I'm not that smart." His comment made me smile, thinking of how I have enjoyed writing poetry with every kind of person imaginable and that speed and intelligence have never been an issue. We can reveal emotion and experience in very simple words if we work from the heart.

The word *therapy* can also be challenging to many. It suggests that something in us needs "fixing," that we are broken, maybe even "crazy." One characteristic of language is that the meanings of words are always changing and original meanings can get lost. We need to remind ourselves that language evolved from nature, the sounds of the creatures, and the flow of water and wind, and that poets not only preserve language, but evolve it. History tells us that therapy comes from the Greek word *therapeia,* which means to *cure through dance, song, poem,* and *drama* (Poplawski, 1994). Characters symbolizing the human condition were able to express what is so difficult to express that effected katharsis, a cleansing of the soul. Through an integration of the catharsis, people gained increased understanding of themselves and others around them. The creative arts were our first therapy. As such, they played a significant role in nourishing souls and expanding understanding of human nature. It is not very different today.

HISTORY OF POETRY THERAPY

The story of poetry as therapy is an old one. An early Inuit poem titled "Magic Words," translated by Edward Field, holds the mystery of language as an early sacred and healing act. I often read this poem to my poetry therapy groups. In part, it reads

> In the very earliest times . . .
> a person could become an animal
> if he wanted to
> and an animal could become a human being . . .
>
> That was a time
> when words were like magic.
> The mind had mysterious powers,
> and a word uttered by chance . . .
> would suddenly come alive
> and what people wanted to happen
> could happen—
> All you had to do was say it.
> Nobody could explain it,
> that's just the way it was.

(Field, 1998)

As this poem suggests, a word could "come alive." The miraculous could occur. We have no way of knowing the results of private rituals where healing is concerned, but Native literature is filled with chants such as "Magic Words to Feel Better," "Magic Words for Hunting Caribou," "Poem to ease birth," "Snake Medicine Poem for a Toothache" (Rothenberg, 1972).

From the beginning, medicine and the arts have been intertwined. In Greek mythology we know that Asclepius, the God of Healing, was the son of Apollo, God of Poetry. Hermes served as messenger between the two worlds to communicate between the gods and humanity. He carried the caduceus, "the winged rod with two serpents intertwined, which has become a symbol of the medical profession" (Poplawski, 1994, p. 75). Poems have also been viewed as carriers of messages from the unconscious to the conscious mind.

In Plato's *Ion,* Socrates defines his magnet chain theory that linked people according to profession by chains. The poet was closest to God, but furthest removed from those who made sense, such as the physician and rhetorician, masters of logic and science.

> . . . all good poets, epic as well as lyric, compose their beautiful poems not by art, but because they are inspired and possessed . . . not by art does the poet sing, but by power divine . . . poets are only interpreters of the Gods . . . (Adler, 1952, p. 144)

Herein lies the mystery of poetry, and perhaps why it has the power to heal. When people are connected to their emotion, they are able to speak a truth outside of reason and come to know and understand another truth to change perception and lift them from darkness.

Dr. J. L. Moreno, founder of psychodrama and noted as the father of group psychotherapy was also interested in poetry as therapy, which he called psychopoetry (Schloss, 1976). Moreno links the actions and words of the medicine man to his theory. He writes of an experience a friend of his encountered with the Pomo Indians near California's West coast. A man felt as if he was dying, having become terrified on encountering something he had never seen before—a wild turkey. With his assistant, the medicine man acted out every detail of the story; playing the role of the turkey, he flew around the sick man who could then perceive the bird as harmless and see that his fears were only a figment of the imagination. "In primitive dramatic rites, the aboriginal performer was not as actor, but a priest . . . like a psychiatrist engaged in saving the tribe, persuading the sun to shine or the rain to fall" (Moreno, 1970, p. 13).

In the late 1950s, Dr. Jack Leedy met Eli Greifer, a New York lawyer and pharmacist who also wrote poetry and believed in its power to help the emotionally disturbed. He volunteered to start a poetry group for patients at Creedmoor State Hospital in New York and in 1963 authored *Principles of Poetry Therapy.* He is attributed with giving poetry therapy its name. Dr. Leedy was so impressed with Greifer, he asked him to work with poetry under his supervision at the Cumberland Hospital in Brooklyn. This was not the first time that poetry had been used for healing in a hospital setting, however. In the 1800s Benjamin Rush "was the first American to recommend reading for the sick and the mentally ill." In 1843, psychiatric patients submitted poems for the Pennsylvania Hospital newspaper *The Illuminator* (Mazza, 1999, p. 5).

Moreno was so encouraged with the work of Leedy and Greifer that he invited them to present panels and demonstrate their work at annual meetings of the American society for group psychotherapy and psychodrama during the 1960s. As more people became interested, the Association for Poetry Therapy (APT) was established in 1969.

In Los Angeles, Dr. Arthur Lerner, a psychologist and poet, had been running poetry therapy groups at Woodview Calabassas Hospital and conducting sessions in poetry therapy under the auspices of UCLA Extension. In 1973, Lerner founded the poetry therapy institute, "the first legally incorporated nonprofit organization devoted to the study and practice of poetry therapy" (Mazza, 1999, p. 7). He also authored, among other books, *Poetry in the Therapeutic Experience* (1978). The National Association for Poetry Therapy (NAPT) was established in 1981 as an outgrowth of Dr. Lerner and Dr. Leedy's early work, along with others. In 1988, I was fortunate to meet Dr. Lerner who invited me to join NAPT and become his student/trainee. I attended several of his groups and meetings before his death in 1998. One of his many talents was his ability to draw the right poem from his mind at the right moment for the right person. His signature lines from a poem by W. H. Auden have become imbedded in the hearts of poetry therapists:

> In the deserts of the heart
> Let the healing fountain start . . .

Dr. Lerner wrote (1997) that the inauguration of the *Journal of Poetry Therapy: The Interdisciplinary Journal of Practice, Theory, Research and Education* (edited by Dr. Nicholas Mazza) was an important milestone in the development of the field. The journal publishes articles about poetry therapy, bibliotherapy, journal therapy, and research in these fields. Another important step occurred in 1980 with the creation of the national federation for biblio/poetry therapy at the initiation of Arleen Hynes and her coworkers. Its purpose is to "uphold advanced standards . . . while developing qualifications and requirements for acceptable professional performance." Through a mentorship program, the federation sets guidelines for training certified poetry therapists for developmental work, and registered poetry therapists for clinical work.

Gilbert Schloss, also influential in the formation of poetry therapy as a dynamic approach to healing, wrote in his book *Psychopoetry* (1976) of the need for research in the field. He posed the following questions:

What is the relationship between an individual's psychological problems and the kind of language and images he uses? Do the symbols and images he uses change as he moves further into therapy? If they do not change, do the meanings of these symbols and images change? Are different kinds of poetry reflective of different psychological disorders? To what extent could an individual's own poetry—or the poetry he responds to most— be utilized as a diagnostics of his psychological problems? (Schloss, 1976, p. 24)

These questions are beginning to be answered in this exciting growing field of therapy. Dr. James W. Pennebaker at the University of Texas in Austin has examined the effectiveness of writing on the physical, emotional, and psychological well being. His research is demonstrating that writing about emotional topics improves the immune system by reducing "stress, anxiety and depression," helps to "improve grades in college," and "aid people in securing new jobs" (Pennebaker, 1990, p. 40). We do not know at this point the specific effect of poetry on a person's well-being, but the National Association for Poetry Therapy has formed a research committee that is beginning ways to develop protocol to explore this work. *The Journal of Poetry Therapy* also publishes studies in this growing field.

POETRY THERAPY IN A RESIDENTIAL
TREATMENT CENTER

While writing a research paper on poetry therapy, I came across an interesting comment: *the schizophrenic sinks in the same waters the enlightened swim* (Murphy, 1979). After becoming licensed as a marriage and family therapist and registered poetry therapist, I decided to test those waters and volunteered to do a poetry therapy group once a week for a month at Sanctuary House, a residential treatment center for those suffering chronic mental illness.

The first poem I read was N. Scott Momaday's "The Delight Song of Tsoai-Talee."

> I am a feather on the bright sky . . .
> I am the hunger of a young wolf . . .
>
> (Momaday, 1983)

I found that the repetition of line beginnings, the strong rhythms and imagery, and the idea that we can be anything we identify with gave the clients comfort. They were excited to talk about their favorite lines and how entertaining it was to think of themselves as something other than a mental health patient.

The concept of simile and metaphor were introduced, naming one thing like another or as another that rises from feeling. I asked them to think about if they ever felt like a feather or horse or hungry wolf? They spoke of their life's struggles, their fears of death, and how good it felt to feel alive in the moment. The poem gave them hope to go on. Then they wrote their own poems that began with "I am," using images and metaphors, of things they had felt one with at some point in their lives.

One client wrote, "I used to be a skunk but now I am a jack rabbit." When they were finished, those who wanted to read it aloud for the gathering could read their poems. We explored a line or two of each poem read, the memory and feelings behind it, and what else it brought up for them. Poetry therapy addresses these facets of poems, not if the poem works. That is addressed in poetry workshops. Poetry therapy never judges a client's response, but is curious about it. A spoken line in response to the poem or question may lead to what clients write. The poems read and written are springboards for exploration and discussion about their lives.

Whereas the group had begun very cautiously and most participants were inhibited and unsure, it ended with great excitement and conversation. "Can we do this again?" I was asked. Fourteen years later I am still working here and just as awed each week to hear clients listen to another poet's words to find their own. In the past years, I have also facilitated groups for hospice clients and the learning disabled. For the purpose of this chapter, however, I will focus on writing groups with clients at the psychiatric residential and day treatment center who have several different diagnoses. Nevertheless, my comments apply, for the most part, to all groups.

Many clients have never written poetry, indeed may not like to write at all. But over the years only a very few have not written. However, their writing is not the most important. What they hear in the presented poems, discussion of these poems, and participation is most significant. They give each other feedback on lines or feelings they heard from each other with which they identify. The other day a client said to me after the group, "I love poetry. It makes me feel normal." Another said, "I feel smart when we talk and write."

On the last day of being a part of the group, after being at the center for almost a year, a young man thanked the group for listening to him all those months. "I have found a new part of myself through writing poetry. I like myself and can face the world again." The comment indicated to me that poetry had brought about a significant change and transformation in that person. He had followed his rhythms. He had gotten in touch with his own healthy thoughts again.

TRAINING IN POETRY THERAPY

The National Association for Poetry Therapy provides several opportunities for education through long distance mentor/supervision programs and training centers. Those interested can log onto their Web site at www.poetrytherapy.org to get information on how to pursue the field further, or phone 1-866-844-NAPT.

I came into the field as a poet first and then received education and licensing as a therapist. Others come into the field as therapists, and fulfill their background in poetry and writing. Some are psychiatrists who want to learn how to work in-depth with poetry. Some are teachers, nurses, and social workers. Some are in business. All those who are drawn to the field of poetry therapy, love poetry, and literature and feel that these art forms have been a catalyst in their own growth process and healing. They want to give to others the satisfying and transformational experience that they have had. Trained poetry therapists work with many populations including adolescents at risk, the elderly, the bereaved, those living with cancer, alcohol and substance abuse clients, the depressed, the developmentally disabled, those suffering HIV/AIDS, trauma victims, sexual abuse survivors, the homeless, and with families. Becoming skilled as a poetry therapist is a valuable journey because it honors what a trainee has already learned and, with a mentor/supervisor, designs an individual training plan that will fulfill his or her goals.

One of the requirements is the practice itself, with groups or individuals who often touch us deeply. Working with an experienced mentor/supervisor teaches the art of working with literature in a holistic way for the purpose of integrating and healing body, mind and spirit. Choosing the right poem is vital, and how a therapist uses that poem with clients is an art that takes time. How closely a therapist *listens* to what a client responds to in a poem, and writes, is key to the process, as well as what the therapist hears that needs valuing and supporting.

The poem is a circle of both intrapersonal and interpersonal communication for growth and so is the mentoring process. As the teacher and the student speak directly to each other about the clients they are working with, each acknowledges the gifts the other has to give. The theory of poetry therapy is integrated with other psychological theories and applied to each situation from which we learn something new. The pebble of the moment dropped in the water expands learning in all directions.

That being said, one of the most beautiful gifts we can give ourselves or another is to write a poem which explodes out of longing or loss or pure joy, with no concern for judgment or condemnation. We can keep the poem in our pocket or purse, and once in a while we can shine a light on it and read it over and over, letting its rhythms soothe us, feeling proud we have spoken the unspeakable, and, if we choose, share it with another person we trust. A child once said to me, "Every time I write a poem, I fall in love with it."

GUIDELINES FOR THE PRACTICE
OF POETRY THERAPY

Poets often wonder when they learn I am a poetry therapist as well as a poet, why everyone thinks that she or he can write a poem. They often ask, "Why do you have to have a special field for poetry therapy?" Lerner (1997, p. 85) pinpoints the issue behind the question when he writes:

> The idea that two fields are combined to form a discipline of a special kind often arouses feelings of territorial rights. Both poetry and therapy have their own history and their own adherents, each with their special ways of looking at and understanding their areas.

The question above demonstrates not only the territoriality of some poets, but also a sincere confusion about how therapeutic process differs from the artistic one. There are as many different ways to write a poem as there are poets and types of poetry, and anytime someone writes a poem, it has therapeutic value. The poet who labors over his or her craft cannot understand how someone could write a poem in 10 minutes and call it a poem. However, in the therapeutic context, this happens again and again. Whether writing poetry for art or therapy, the same techniques apply: use of simile, metaphor, and other figurative speech; use of rhythm, repetition, and word choice; and use of imagery and form. How these techniques are presented, however, is quite different in the therapeutic model.

The goals of a poetry therapy session are to increase self-esteem and positive self-regard, to understand self and others, to discover new parts of self, to gain greater coping skills, to know the self as a greater part of the whole, and to improve "reality orientation" (Hynes & Hynes-Berry, 1994). A poem is selected based on its accessibility, clarity of language, strong theme as well as emotions. Another essential element is that the poem must resonate with the mood and/or situation of the group or individual. This is called the *isoprinciple,* a term also used in music therapy for the same purpose. Jack Leedy (1985) says that "the poem becomes symbolically an understanding of someone with whom they can share their despair" (p. 82). The poem becomes a personification, in a way, of a person who has had similar experiences as the reader. Adams and Rojcewicz (2003), in *The Healing Fountain,* further explain that the selected poem "should not be excessively negative or glorify suicide or anti-social behavior . . . but (chosen) for its usefulness as a tool for awareness, self-discovery, and therapeutic change."

One time, while working with an individual client who did not particularly care for poetry, I spontaneously pulled out the poem "Wild Geese" by Mary Oliver. The mother of the client, age 40, had passed away when the client was 14 years old. Over the two months we had been working together, the client claimed that she was well over the loss of her mother and that her stepmother, age 50, had taken her mother's place. The issue we were working on that day was that she never seemed to get anything right. I asked her to read the poem. When she came to the lines near the end, "The world . . . calls to you like the wild geese, harsh and exciting . . . announcing your place in the family of things" she burst into sobs saying this poem was about her mother. When I asked her how that was so, she said, "She loved geese. Where we lived they flew all the time and she would always run out and wave to them." Quite accidentally I had selected the right poem for the moment. This breakthrough allowed her to begin deep grieving work that had kept her from her potential for so many years.

In *Biblio/Poetry Therapy the Interactive Process: A Handbook* (1994), Arleen McCarty Hynes and Mary Hynes-Berry outline the following four steps, which are widely used in the process of poetry therapy: recognition, examination, juxtaposition, and application to self.

Step One: Recognition. Something in the material presented "'engages' the participant," grabs their attention, "stops wandering thoughts, opens imagination." Oftentimes after a first reading, a response will pop out such as "I love this poem," or "this is exactly how I feel." Perhaps the poem communicates something the client has experienced. Feeling bonded with the poet, there can be an immediate catharsis, if the poem is a "someone" with whom they share their sorrow (Hynes & Hynes-Berry, 1994, p. 45).

Step Two: Examination. It is advisable to read a selection twice: the first time to see what is there, and the second time to feel more. After responding to initial reactions general questions are asked, such as:

Where do you find yourself in the poem? What phrases or lines appeal to you? What do these lines remind you of? Do they bring up any memories? Are you surprised by anything in the poem? Rather than discussion of what the poem *means*, it centers around what it means to the client.

Often the therapist might ask whether there is anything confusing about the poem. This gives valuable information. The whole time examination is going on, the therapist might invite the client to talk about his or her responses. Is there anything the client doesn't like about the poem? Would she or he end the poem differently? These questions often bring about a lively discussion and from that participants will often say something that is filled with emotion. Often I write a client's words down and read back as a poem. The client may hold the paper and look at it as if it were a mirror, startled at the image as if seeing him or her self for the first time, or being seen. I never keep these poems. Clients fold them next to their hearts, where they belong.

Step Three: Juxtaposition. Putting old ideas next to new ones in a poem, following examination, can change a client's thinking and feeling about a situation, the self, or another person. For instance, if a poem speaks of how every person is valuable no matter who they are or what they do, clients in a treatment center, thinking they are wasting their lives, might conclude after discussion that the work they are doing healing themselves is just as important as having a job or raising a child. They are raising themselves, learning to live in a world that "offers itself" to their "imagination," thinking of Mary Oliver's poem.

Step Four: Application to Self. A client lastly needs to integrate what she or he has learned from the first three steps. She or he must learn to talk differently about him or her self, and think about applying newly formed concepts to behaviors and attitudes. For instance, if a client has thought of himself as "stupid" or a "loser" but through discussion of a poem realizes he or she is bright and has much to offer others through his or her opinions, he or she will feel empowered to change his or her life.

It would be helpful to ask a client, for instance, how will he or she "rename" him or her self? What steps can he or she take to improve his or her behavior? Is he or she willing to change? How can he or she use his or her intelligence and imagination in a new way? Oftentimes, there is some *resolution* within the poem that a client can use to help him or her decide to change his or her course. In short, the whole experience can give a client new *meaning* which can be a step toward hope and healing. For example, a client wrote the following poem after being in the poetry therapy group for a year.

"Wish Granted"

Once upon a time so wild
I used drugs to tame my child
Voodoo could not make me mild
And so my soul had been defiled

But then one day the curse did lift
Sobriety became a gift
No more would I sink and drift
Further down an endless rift

Nicholas Mazza (1999, p. 17) proposed a slightly different variation to the process of poetry therapy, but it contains the same steps:

1. The receptive/prescriptive component involving the introduction of literature into therapy
2. The expressive/creative component involving the use of client writing and therapy
3. The symbolic/ceremonial component involving the use of metaphors, rituals and storytelling

POETRY THERAPY GROUP GUIDELINES

When a poetry therapy group is being formed, it is essential, as in any group work, that safety be established. Confidentiality must be explained. No one may judge another's writing as being a "good" or "bad" poem. Rather they are asked to talk about lines in the writing that spoke to them, what had *meaning* for them, or share briefly an experience they had that is similar to the one shared. Only the facilitator may make therapeutic comments or questions, such as "it sounds like you are having a very difficult time. Would you care to talk more about what it was like when . . .?" A group member may ask someone to read their poem, or certain lines of their poem, again. When a new member comes into the group, clients often enjoy telling them how the group works.

Many poetry therapists engage the group or client with the theme of the poem before reading it. For instance, if Robert Frost's poem "The Road Not Taken" is to be explored, it might be discussed if anyone has ever had difficulty making a decision or if they have ever regretted a decision. This helps to channel thought before the process begins. Some therapists like to do a "warm up" writing exercise before the main writing begins. Considering the Robert Frost poem, a therapist might ask them to briefly describe a favorite road they have experienced.

With psychiatric groups, I will often lead a group "oral" poem that comes from a sentence stem in the poem, which may trigger ideas to write about. For instance, if the poem is about fear, we might begin "I feel afraid when . . ." With groups that have difficulty writing, I will often write down what they say, type it up, and bring it in the next week, which gives them great pleasure and a deep sense of being valued. Lauren Slater, in her book *Welcome to My Country* (1996), writes of a client in a similar environment, who said after seeing his words typed up, "You typed it up, you typed it up . . . Hello, my mother. My words." And then he began to cry. Slater (1996) goes on to say how she wanted to hug him "as his mother might have, but there is only so much hurt you can heal" (p. 111). After typing, I bind the clients' poems in their personal three-ring folders. When I asked a client one day, as he held his book close to his heart, what that felt like, he wept, "I finally feel like I am somebody." He was a young man who had never written, but spoke in poetry. Words that usually buzzed around in his head with no order were written down and given shape. To be valued as a writer gave him an identity other than a mentally ill person. It gave him hope in himself.

Sometimes the healing moment occurs in the interactions that clients have with each other as a result of their written poems. One day in poetry group I had been asked to read the residents their treatment rights. I suggested each begin a line with "I have a right to . . ." thinking of their every day lives. Thoughts came forth like "I have a right to breathe," "I have the right to eat healthy food." One male client burst forth, "I have the right to take a gun and shoot myself." Another client, who had come to group intermittently over several months, but who had never written or spoken much, abruptly spoke up with gentility and compassion, "And I have the right to take it from you." The quiet that settled in the room bore deeply into everyone. Many had experienced suicide attempts, even this woman. In that moment, when you could hear only breath, it was as if the poem with all its process steps came together at once. The young man cried, feeling the care of another group member who had not noticed him before. The female client, grieving the loss of her own child who was taken from her, could experience being the young man's mother. Silence in such moments is one of the most important guidelines, for it is a healing presence, a warmth that shifts perception.

After clients are given 10 to 15 minutes to write their own poems, they are given the opportunity to read them, if they choose. It is important not to push this, for what they have written may feel too personal in the group setting. I like to collect the poems when given permission, read them, and write comments on a sticky note. I tell the group member how the poem affects me, what I see there and what insights I notice. I do not evaluate the poem as a teacher would. I suggest what actions the clients might take toward caring for themselves, or what they might want to remember. When people know their work is read and heard, it is a way to "hold" the client. Some clients have said to me that it is the "sticky notes" they value most of all.

HEALING ELEMENTS OF POETRY

Often I am asked how to respond to client poems, if saying "that's really good" or "wonderful" is not helpful in a therapy environment. To explain this, we only need to look at the healing elements of poetry: the form or shape of poetry itself, the metaphor, the metamessage, the words chosen, and the sounds of the words together (alliteration and assonance). These elements in association with each other carry the weight of many feelings and messages, creating a link from the secret internal world to external reality.

Another healing component of poetry is its shape. Because it has a border, as opposed to prose, the form itself is a safety net. If we feel strong emotions, there is a built-in sense that the poem will contain them. We will not run off the page. It is a form of control. I often ask clients to draw a box in the center of the page and write the words inside.

Metamessages of words in a poem have a powerful ability to heal. Metamessage implies the ability to carry several messages in one line that "strike at deeper levels of awareness than overt messages" (Murphy, 1979, p. 69). This is because we learned language from the tones of our mother's voice and the emotions it conveyed. Through the capacity to convey many messages, clients are able to experience merging as well as individuation and separation. The poem allows for a trial separation and then a return to the therapist for merging and "refueling" through the therapist's understanding of the poem. If the therapist says she appreciates a particular metaphor and how the words flow, the client feels loved. In reading a poem aloud, the client may become caught up in his own rhythms and feel caressed.

Multi-messages are also carried in the sounds of the words themselves. Many years ago one of my acting teachers quoted Constantin Stanislavski who said "the vowels are the rivers of the soul and the consonants are the banks." I like to think of this, when listening to clients read their poems. Language is its own safety valve. Low tones of mourning can be coupled with the hiss of "s" words or the plosive nature of "p" sounds.

Robert Frost's well-known poem, "The Road Not Taken," ends:

> Two roads diverged in a wood, and I—
> I took the one less traveled by,
> And that has made all the difference.

These lines often come up in a group as members flow in and out of the residential and day treatment center. If clients are new to the program, and young, they often complain about being "sent" there. If older, they feel despair at suffering for years with their illness, one they did not choose for their life. The poem brings up issues about choices they can make for themselves while they are in treatment.

In response to the discussion of this poem, a female client who has been in and out of the group for about four years wrote the following poem.

"This Day"

What road do I take when
The sun arises over the hill?
What course do I take
When it lights this side of the world?

Or, even the night before,
Falling into a rhythmic breath
To hold me all the night long,
With many a dream to sustain me?

Do I turn left or right?
Walk, bike, drive?
Frolic, skip or run?
Work, read, write or draw?

What are my thoughts?
Positive, negative, doubting, or strong?
Do I need to focus?
Or, does God do the guiding?

I stop now to see the flowers,
yet know not what the day will bring,
Because all days may change our plans.
And night always settles in, whether
expected or not.

After she read this poem, the group members spontaneously applauded. One female client responded, "That's so good." When I asked if she could say why, she replied by saying that it made her "feel good." She then directed her comment to the writer of the poem, saying she liked how she moved in all those different ways down the road. I pointed out to the writer that even though she was unsure whether her road for the day was the right one, she made the best of it by considering her choices. Another participant pointed out how days were unpredictable. That morning she woke up depressed, but the poem made her feel happy, because there was sun in it.

The client who wrote the poem suffers schizophrenia. She often has loose thought associations and this was one of her more focused poems. I told her how I liked that she paused to look at the flowers.

"They help," she replied. The image, one of beauty, shows increased awareness of the world around her, and that she can draw on nature as well as reading and writing to help her get through the day.

The lines: "Do I need to focus?/Or, does God do the guiding?" were interesting to me. "My experience of your poem is that you seem happy moving on a road God has helped guide you toward. Is it something like that?" Clients enjoy the therapist asking about the meaning behind their poem. They can then correct it, if the therapist is wrong. It also helps clarify their own meaning, which may not occur to them when they are writing. When they give an opinion, it helps them to know the "I." In this way, poetry therapy builds ego strength. The client's response was that when she worried too much, she would ask God to help silence her thoughts. I then asked her if she would talk more about the last line, about night settling in. She said that she could not. Another client suggested what it meant to him was that some days are so long you think they will never end. Yet another said that night came too soon.

This example gives some sense of how a poem can be talked about in a touching way, moving away from the evaluative judgments to which we have been so conditioned. The therapist herself can look at the poem for the layers of meaning within the sounds of words and between the words. Throughout the poem the schizophrenic client displays anxiety with her questions, but at the same time she enjoys herself in the words selected. She asks whether she should "frolic, skip, or run," not crawl or drag. The rhythm bounces. By the last stanza, however, the lines are longer and more lyrical. Even when plans change, she can hold some beauty in her heart that she has perceived during the day. When she mentions "change," the language becomes crisper. The "t" sounds express some anger about the not knowing, but also contain confusion. Looking at poetry through language, rhythm, form, and metaphor help frame questions to process the client's meaning more deeply and create an understanding we might not otherwise have.

CASE STUDY

A client who names her writing self Melody Atrabili, meaning to her, "the song of sadness," wrote and published an article about the importance of writing poetry in her life from the age of 17 until she left the sanctuary of psychiatric treatment centers three years ago. The public Melody was an accomplished honors student, top runner, officer of many clubs in school, and valedictorian of her high school class. She thought this was her path to happiness because it made others happy to see her doing so well.

However, she thought of herself as "lazy, selfish, mean, stupid . . . and the odd one out." Over the years she had received multiple diagnoses including major depression, borderline personality disorder, schizo-affective disorder, Asperger's disorder and most recently, depression and anxiety. In her article published in *The Journal of the California Alliance for the Mentally Ill* (Strohman, 1998), she writes:

> I wished for someone to help look out for me when I couldn't ask for what I needed or even figure out what I needed. . . . However, through my poems, I began to have awarenesses about my illness. My poems were teaching me.

Over time, Melody shared her early poems with me, those that she had written in high school, and usually she shared the poems she wrote for three years in the poetry therapy group. In June of 2001 she wanted to meet individually for a few sessions before she took off to continue with her studies, working toward a PhD in food chemistry. We decided to assess the content of her poems to see if they had changed over time, her feelings about her poetry, and if writing had helped her.

At our first session Melody referred to the sticky notes I wrote on her poems "I really treasure them. I can tell you read my poems and you understand what I was saying or the point I was trying to make." She then asked me to re-read the following poem.

"I Write Poetry"

I write poetry
but I don't write pretty poetry
not a handful of daisies freshly picked
that you grabbed on the way home for your mother
not warm fireplaces that you can curl up before

in your easy chair with your cat
not ballerinas dancing gracefully
in pastel colored tutus, now bowing low before
  the audience
not intricately designed watercolors
that bathe your eyes in light shades of dew
but not snakes that lie at the foot of your bed
ready to strike either
I write poems of slow moving streams
that quickly morph into rapids and treacherous waterfalls
I write poems of boats on a sea
in a torrential and windy downpour
I write poems of puzzles
with places where no piece could fit
I write poems threatening to overturn the status quo
with a see-saw and a bucket of mud
I write poems of packages tied up with ribbons
but the ribbons have jumpy ends and tangle with others
  of their kind
I write poems of a truth at the moment
one that is clear or quite hard to see
I write poems as sharp and jagged as shards of glass
and as easy to see through as tattered silk
I write poems
but they are not all concise, elegant, and delightful
they are not pretty

Because this is one of Melody's favorite poems, I asked her what
in the poem satisfied her. She talked about how in high school people
were always saying she did not live up to her potential. In response to
this, Melody would run three or four miles if asked to run one. With a
poem, however, she never put this pressure on herself, which is why
she often writes poems about poems. The poem is like someone who
understands that "pretty things" exist with things that are not, a notion that captures both warring sides of her psyche but one that is
blended in the safety net of the poem, which eases confusion. Oppos-
ing words capture the forces in her life: easy chair, cat, fireplace, in
juxtaposition with snakes and treacherous waterfalls, shards of glass

"as easy to see through as tattered silk." The metamessage is that her imagination is fueled with the power of writing, and through it she comes to know and accept herself, not her "mental illness." She is capable of "cheering herself on" just as she has others.

In another session, she pointed out a poem written in 1996, when she was very suicidal, written with the lower case "i" to delineate her small self who wants to evaporate. The pronoun "we" in the title refers to herself and a friend, also suicidal. He wanted to "touch" her, but she didn't want him to. "I have to live so I won't hurt other people," she said.

"what we said"

i don't feel like
living today
i'll buy a gun
a great big one
we'll leave this world
it is no fun

but think about
the simple touch
which with understanding
can mean so much

if the choice is mine alone
then i could simply choose to die
but if it would hurt another's heart
i'll change my mind and choose to try.

The last stanza, she explained, is about her being a peacemaker. She never wanted to leave her work undone or friends in disarray no matter how badly she felt. She needed to keep trying to live.

On the day of Melody's last session she talked about how poems help her identify her feelings, and that is most rewarding. "If I have a feeling and I don't know a *reason*, I have trouble identifying and accepting that feeling." Her poetry often helps her find a reason, it seems. In one of her last poems she writes:

don't worry
i could not attempt suicide now
i do not have enough time
however, i am almost compelled
to tempt fate by slashing my arms with a razor
or casing out buildings to climb up high
and sit and ponder life
or to walk slowly across
the street at a yellow light
as usual i keep running
as usual i can't escape

I was concerned that she still wanted to harm herself, and questioned from what could she not escape. Looking further, I understood that her goals would keep her moving forward, that she would "ponder" and "walk slow" and that she would also "keep running." She could not escape her determination to keep going. She could not escape life.

Perhaps one of the best things poetry as therapy has to offer is that through emotional release, empathic listening, and validation, the client finds her voice and speaking it, builds resistance to life's challenges so that she can continue. That, for some, is a miracle in itself. In the exchange of searching for meaning behind the words, there is always the surprise of the poem, itself a light in the darkness.

REFERENCES

Adams, K. & Rojcewicz, S. (2003). Mindfulness on the journey ahead. In G.G. Chavisand & L.L. Weisberger (Eds.), *The healing fountain: Poetry therapy for life's journey.* St. Cloud Press, MN: North Star Press.

Adler, M.J. (Assoc. Ed). (1952). Ion. In *The dialogues of Plato, Great Books of the Western World,* Vol. 7. Chicago, IL: Encyclopaedia Britannica, Inc.

Barks, C. (tr.) (1992). *Naked song.* North Reading, MA: Maypop Books.

Chavis, G.G. & Weisberger, L.L. (Eds.). (2003). *The healing fountain: Poetry therapy for life's journey.* St. Cloud, MN: North Star Press.

Field, E. (Ed.). (1998). Magic words. In *Frieze for a temple of love* (pp. 32-33). Santa Rosa, CA: Black Sparrow Press.

Hynes, A.M. & Hynes-Berry, M. (1994). *Biblio/Poetry therapy: The interactive process.* St. Cloud, MN: North Star Press.

Kemplar, N.Z. (2003). Finding our voice through poetry and psychotherapy. *Journal of Poetry Therapy, 16*(4), 217-220.

Leedy, J.J. (Ed.). (1969). *Poetry therapy.* Philadelphia: J.B. Lippincott Company.

Leedy, J.J. (Ed.). (1985). *Poetry as healer: Mending the troubled mind.* New York: Vanguard.

Lerner, A. (Ed.). (1978, 1994). *Poetry in the therapeutic experience.* St. Louis, MO: MMB Music, Inc.

Lerner, A. (1997). A look at poetry therapy. *The Arts in Psychotherapy, 24*(1), 81-89.

Mazza, N. (1999). *Poetry therapy: Interface of the arts and psychology.* Boca Raton, FL: CRC Press.

Momaday, N.S. (1983). The delight song of Tsoai-Talee. In J. Bruchac, (Ed.). *Songs from this earth on Turtle's Back.* New York: The Greenfield Review Press.

Moreno, J.L. (1970). *Psychodrama,* Vol. 1. New York: Beacon House, Inc.

Murphy, J.M. (1979). The therapeutic use of poetry. In Jules Masserman (Ed.). *Current psychiatric therapies,* Vol. 18 (65-72). New York: Grune & Stratton, Inc.

National Association for Poetry Therapy. 777 E. Atlantic Avenue, #243, Delray Beach, FL 33483. www.poetrytherapy.org.

National Association for Poetry Therapy (circa 1996). *What is poetry therapy?* Brochure printed by the National Association for Poetry Therapy.

Oliver, M. (1993). Wild geese. *New and selected poems.* Boston: Beacon Press.

Pennebaker, J. (1990). *Opening up: The healing power of expressing emotions.* New York: Guilford Press.

Poplawski, T. (1994). Schizophrenia and the soul. *The Quest,* August, 74-79.

Rothenberg, J. (1972). *Shaking the pumpkin: Traditional poetry of the Indian North Americas.* New York: Doubleday & Co., Inc.

Schloss, Gt. (1976). *Psychopoetry.* New York: Grosset & Dunlap.

Slater, L. (1996). *Welcome to my country.* New York: Random House, p. 111.

Strohman, D. (1998 December, 28). I lead a double life. *The Journal of the California Alliance for the Mentally Ill, 9*(2), 75-77.

Witherspoon, G. (1977). *Language and art in the Navajo universe.* Ann Arbor: University of Michigan Press.

Chapter 5

Art Therapy

Laura A. Cherry

In its broadest definition, art is the human act of expression through creativity. A work of art displays elements of form and beauty and indicates to the observer the understanding of those elements as they are perceived by the work's creator. Through his or her work the artist communicates feelings and perceptions concerning a personal, physical, and psychological self, and is able to convey viewpoints about society and the world in which he or she lives. The artist may choose to communicate in a manner in which the message is obvious or occult, symbolic or realistic, and the observer of the work is free to react to that message as it fits in with his or her own frame of reference. Art in all of its many forms is the method of communication that transcends all languages, embraces all cultures, and on occasion allows those who have no voice to express themselves. It is the component of communication inherent in all art forms that has led to the emergence of several therapies (dance, music, psychodrama) that are based on the arts. The focus of this chapter on art therapy is on the process of aiding clients in the therapeutic creation of images based on clients' thoughts, feelings, experiences, wishes, and fears. Art therapists work with a variety of populations both as part of teams or as private practitioners. They work in art studios, clinics, correctional facilities, drug treatment facilities, halfway houses, hospitals (both medical and psychiatric), outpatient facilities, residential treatment facilities, schools, senior care facilities, shelters, universities, and colleges. This chapter will include an overview of the field and history of art therapy, basic

Introduction to Alternative and Complementary Therapies
© 2008 by The Haworth Press, Taylor & Francis Group. All rights reserved.
doi:10.1300/5987_05

art therapy approaches, a highlight of research that documents the effectiveness of art therapy, and guidelines for practicing art therapy. The benefits of art therapy extend to both children and adults; a case study involving a six-year-old boy is presented in this chapter.

DESCRIPTION OF MODALITY

Art therapy is "a professional discipline that is a synthesis of psychology, art, and other social science and humanities disciplines" (Lark, 2001, p. 32). Art therapy is the process of creating art in order to increase awareness of self and others, cope with symptoms, stress, and traumatic experiences, and enjoy the life affirming pleasures of making art. The American Art Therapy Association (AATA) defines art therapy as a human service profession that utilizes art media, images, the creative art process, and patient/client responses to the created art production as a reflection of an individual's development, abilities, personality, interests, concerns, and conflicts (AATA, 2005). Art therapy practice is based on knowledge of human developmental and psychological theories that are implemented in the full spectrum of models of assessment and treatment as means of reconciling emotional conflicts, fostering self-awareness, developing social skills, managing behavior, solving problems, reducing anxiety, aiding reality orientation, and increasing self-esteem.

At the center of art therapy is creativity and symbolic representation yet the client does not need to be a trained artist to benefit from this approach to therapy. Even the client who has difficulty with verbal expression is often able to discuss his or her artwork in order to explain the images he or she has created. The art therapist does not interpret the client's art expression, but instead encourages the client to share with him or her the meanings of the images produced. As the artwork evolves throughout the course of treatment, it is possible for the client and therapist to visually review any changes in the client's image-making and its content and for both client and therapist to assess how much progress has been made during their therapeutic relationship. The ideas, feelings, and symbols depicted in the client's work become objectified and accessible through imagery that is now separate from them, allowing for reflective distance so that the client can then respond emotionally to the image he or she has created. Images in art therapy are often "regarded as a kind of mirror which reflects, through free associations, what is taking place in the unconscious" (Naumberg, 1966, p. 7).

The Expressive Therapies Continuum (ETC), a conceptual art therapy model, identified and developed by Kagin and Lusebrink (1978), provides a structure and a system for the facilitation of art making in art therapy and includes in its theoretical basis the role of the therapist, client, and the art medium chosen by the client during the therapeutic intervention. The ETC is a four-level developmental continuum that becomes progressively more complex. The lowest level of the continuum is the *kinesthetic-sensory level*. A client working at the kinesthetic dimension of this level is involved in an exploration of materials and motor movements and the release of energy such as he or she might experience when flattening and rolling clay. A client involved in the sensory dimension of this level explores tactile qualities and focuses on inner sensations with minimal reflective distance on his or her part. At the kinesthetic-sensory level, art making is physical with minimal thought given to the final product. An example of art produced at the kinesthetic sensory level would be the creation of an art piece using finger paints and in which minimal direction is given to the client. The next level on the ETC continuum is the *perceptual-affective level*. The perceptual dimension of this level emphasizes form and concrete image creation and focuses on the structural qualities found in the client's artwork such as "defining boundaries, differentiating form, and striving to achieve an appropriate representation for an inner or external experience" (Lusebrink, 1990, p. 93). At the perceptual-affective level, art making is literal in its meaning and represents the interaction between perception and affect. Structured media (such as wood) that are solid and definite in form are used at the perceptual-affective level to help evoke inner organization and stability for the client. The therapist assesses the client along the perceptive-affective dimension by observing his or her artwork, how the client expresses feelings and moods, and the client's use of color, allowing the client to reflect "the emotions expressed and released through the interaction with the media" (Lusebrink, 1990, p. 20). The client is encouraged to identify and explain what feelings are provoked by the images he or she has created. An example of art created at the perceptual-affective level would include creating images using only colors and shapes to identify feelings and moods. The next level on the continuum is the *cognitive-symbolic level*. The cognitive dimension incorporates concept formulation, abstraction, and verbal self-instruction while the symbolic dimension incorporates intuitive and self-oriented concept formation and abstraction. The cognitive level focuses on logical thinking. The symbolic level focuses on the formation of symbols and symbolic expression of meaning as a method of problem-solving leading to insight and emotional growth (Lusebrink, 1990). The final dimension of the ETC is the *creative synthesis level,* which is the act of creative expression that leads to a sense of closure and/or joy. The creative experience can happen on any and all of the levels of the ETC, and is evident when the client experiences a new level of creativity, understanding, and insight.

Art media parallel the dimensions of the ETC. Generally, fluid media (e.g., watercolors, wet clay, chalk pastels, finger paints) are seen as kinesthetic and sensory whereas more controlled media (e.g., pencils, felt tip makers, cut paper collage, colored pencils) are seen as cognitive and symbolic. Fluid materials are considered "easier to manipulate but harder to control because they are watery (such as paints) or powdery (such as chalk pastels)" (Malchiodi, 1998, p. 84). The more controlled or resistive media enable the client to be precise and detailed (Malchiodi, 1998). Understanding the role of the media and the desired outcomes of the use of media enables the art therapist to identify art materials that will stimulate desired client development. If the client has difficulty in accessing his or her feelings, the therapist may seek to advance the client from a cognitive-symbolic (thinking) dimension to a perceptual-affective (feeling) dimension. The ETC is a model that can be used in conjunction with all of the various theoretical approaches. It provides a map for navigating through the art therapy experiences regardless of the theoretical approach.

HISTORY

Hans Prinzhorn is credited as the instigator of art work within clinical settings. Prinzhorn, a German psychiatrist, published *The Artistry of the Mentally Ill* (1922/1972), which displayed the artwork of insane asylum patients from many areas throughout Europe. His work was the catalyst for the use of art in psychiatric settings. Following Prinzhorn's discovery that the use of art could be therapeutic, Margaret Naumberg began to delineate the process that became known as art therapy. In the 1930s, under Naumberg's guidance, art therapy became a clearly identified profession. It was also during this time that art educators discovered the benefits of "free and spontaneous art expression of children [which] represented both emotional and symbolic communication" (www.arttherapy.org). In the 1940s, while working at the Walden School and then later at a psychiatric hospital, Naumberg again saw evidence that the artwork of the children and adult patients were symbolic representations of their unconscious. In *Dynamically Oriented Art Therapy: Its Principles and Practice* (1966), Naumberg described art therapy as a form of psychotherapy that encouraged the use of "symbolic communication between the patient and the therapist" (p. 1). Naumberg emphasized an art-in-therapy model as she encouraged her clients to "draw spontaneously and to associate to their pictures" (Wadeson, 1980, p. 13).

Edith Kramer, who worked primarily with children, began writing about her experiences using art at the Psychoanalytic Institute in Prague. In the 1930s, Kramer worked with refugee children from Nazi Germany. It was during this period that she observed artwork that evidenced the conflict the children were experiencing. Kramer, who moved to the United States in 1938 in an attempt to avoid the Nazis, developed the theory that the artistic creative process was healing and supported the idea of art as a therapy modality. "She emphasized the integrative and healing properties to the creative process itself which does not require verbal reflection" (Wadeson, 1980, p. 13). Kramer emphasized the art as therapy model. She conceived art therapy as "primarily a means of supporting the ego, fostering the development of a sense of identity and promoting maturation in general" (Junge, 1994, p. 34). Kramer viewed the role of the art therapist as a guide or a helper in emphasizing the importance of the unconscious or preconscious in the development of images and symbols (Drachnik, 1995).

In the 70 years or so since Edith Kramer began her work, a number of individuals have been instrumental to the progress of art therapy as a therapeutic modality and profession. Lowenfeld, who coined the phrase "art education therapy," published *Creative and Mental Growth* (1947), which describes children's art development. Lowenfeld observed that the color, line, details, and placement symbolically represents the child's environment and enables the child to express his or her psychological perceptions (Drachnik, 1995). Also in 1947, John Buck designed and published the "House-Tree-Person" (HTP) test that has become a classic art therapy assessment and intervention. The HTP test was developed as a nonverbal intelligence test that evolved into a personality test (Rowe et al., 1993). The HTP helps the clinician to obtain information about the client's sensitivity, maturity, flexibility, efficiency, degree of personality integration, and interaction with their environment (Knapp, 1992). Buck believed that "certain definite and unmistakable signs of underlying psychosis revealed themselves" (Rowe et al., 1993, p. 430) in these drawings and that they were valuable diagnostic material and quickly became used by psychologists because the clients' cooperation visibly improved when permitted to draw. It is also noted that having mental patients draw was not an original idea and it had appeared in literature Buck perused prior to his creation of the HTP.

The client is instructed to complete the HTP using the following script:

> Take one of these pencils please. I want you to draw me as good a picture of a house as you can. You may erase as much as you like, it will not be counted against you. You may take as long as you wish. Just draw me as good a house as you can. (Knapp, 1992, p. 24)

The client is then asked a series of questions about the drawing. The above steps are then repeated for the tree and person drawings. The client is then asked to complete all three drawings again using eight crayons with the same questions being asked after each drawing.

In subsequent years, the field progressed quickly. Myra Levick directed the first graduate level art therapy program in 1967 at Hahnemann Hospital and the Medical College in Philadelphia. At Hahnemann, a group of art therapists agreed to form a national art therapy organization for professional art therapists: the American Art Therapy Association. There are currently 28 graduate level programs approved by the AATA in the United States.

From the late 1950s through the early 1980s, art therapists published important books and articles adding to the knowledge base of the field. Betensky (1973), Gantt and Schmal (1974), Jones (1983), Kramer (1958, 1971), Kwiatkowska (1962), Landgarten (1981), Levick (1967), Naumberg (1966), Rhyne (1973), Rubin (1978), Ulman (1975), and Wadeson, Durkin, and Perach (1989) have all contributed significantly to the progress of the profession.

ART THERAPY APPROACHES

There are a number of art therapy approaches that can be utilized based on the target population and the education and school of thought of the clinician. In broad terms, art therapy is divided into five major approaches: art AS therapy, cognitive-behavioral, developmental, humanistic, and psychoanalytic/psychodynamic. A survey conducted by the AATA indicated that many art therapists use a combination of approaches in their daily practices and consider their approaches to art therapy "eclectic." Most art therapists shift their approaches as the situation or client requires in order to use the approach that is most efficacious.

Art AS Therapy

Unlike the other approaches to art therapy that follow, "art AS therapy" is the simple act of making art as a form of therapy. Although this modality is the foundation for other art therapy approaches, art AS therapy does not seek as other approaches do to change thoughts or behaviors, stimulate development, encourage autonomy, evaluate visual symbols, or to evaluate the therapeutic process. Rather, it considers that it is the properties of art itself and the process of art making that are therapeutic. Practitioners who follow the art AS therapy model rely on the power of creativity and the making of art to enhance individual functioning. "In this approach, neither the artwork nor the therapeutic relationships was analyzed. Full confidence was placed in the inherent properties of art making to be therapeutic within the therapy setting" (Lark, 2001, p. 21). Art AS therapy is used as a way to support the ego, to foster individual growth, and to encourage self-expression in the client. Therapists who use the art AS therapy approach to client intervention focus on the self-expression and self-recognition of the client and accept and encourage all artwork produced by the client.

If we define as art any kind of formed expression, regardless of the level of talent, skill, or mental age, that has some degree of inner consistency, and again within the limitations of the [person's] capacities, a certain evocative power, we can usually decide without too much hesitation whether or not the goal of art has been reached in a [person's] pictures. (Kramer, 1971, p. 50)

The emphasis in art AS therapy, according to Edith Kramer (1971), is on the art and the art making in therapy and on the belief that there is healing inherent in the creation of art and in the creative process itself. The art therapist, therefore, makes the art and art experiences available to the client and acts as a guide or support as the client works through conflicts. "Although art expression cannot directly resolve conflict, it can provide a place where new attitudes and feelings can be expressed and tried out" (Malchiodi, 1998, p. 36). The art therapist should not intervene to alter the clients' image or intent but only assist in the art making when the client appears to struggle with expression. Assistance may be given by the therapist to a client who is physically unable to perform certain actions or who may, unless assisted, be unable to complete a piece of art without danger of breakage.

The catharthic act of creation to facilitate self-expression and the emergence of feelings is supported by the use of art AS therapy. Catharsis frequently occurs as clients experience for themselves the accepting environment provided by the art therapist. The "art processes are a function of creativity, which is therefore central within art therapy" (Dalley et al., 1987, p. 5). The creativity involved in making art is an act that turns feelings, often unconscious, into a concrete form with conscious access. Problematic issues or conflicts are transformed into rational and understandable forms. These issues or conflicts are then re-experienced, resolved, and integrated into the psyche. Each client's art is unique, as are the personal experiences of that individual making art a form of communication that the client can use to connect the meaning of the image produced to his or her own life situation.

As a therapeutic tool, the art form, unique to the individual, provides the focus for discussion, analysis, and self evaluation, and as it is concrete, acts as a record of this activity which cannot be denied, erased, or forgotten. It also survives in time and so is an index of and comparison between past and present. (Dalley, 1984, p. xiv)

Cognitive-Behavioral Art Therapy

Cognitive-behavioral art therapy is a combination of two related approaches. The cognitive approach in art therapy is based on the theory that thoughts and emotions are cognitive means to know, to understand, and to organize information (*American Heritage Dictionary of the English Language,* 2000). Images, such as those created in art therapy, are representations of this information. In a behavioral approach, one seeks to treat and assess reasons for problematic behaviors. Problematic behaviors are seen as the result of environmental and situational determinants and not from faulty cognitions. Faulty cognitions are addressed using the cognitive approach.

Using the cognitive approach to art therapy, the art therapist seeks to identify, develop, and evaluate a client's cognitive skills as they become evident in the artwork and art activities of the client. The art therapist uses art and art activities as an avenue for cognitive growth and any art activity that facilitates problem-solving or conflict resolution is beneficial. Rosal (1992) indicates that there are four major characteristics of cognitive-behavioral art therapy: (1) art is a cognitive activity, (2) art can help change cognitive distortions, (3) mental images can be used therapeutically to affect behavioral chances, and (4) art can help individuals to gain self-control (Rosal, 1992, p. 170). Through the experience of cognitive art therapy, the client "explores emotions as well as thoughts, seeks to ease tensions, and build self-confidence" (Silver, 1987, p. 233). The goals of the cognitive component of cognitive-behavioral art therapy include (1) assisting the client to problem solve through art experiences, (2) helping the client to gain control over feelings, and (3) assessing the cognitive component of problematic behaviors. In order to facilitate these goals and reduce client anxiety, the therapist often utilizes relaxation techniques in combination with art therapy. The focus of behavioral art therapy is to eliminate undesired behaviors or symptoms. Therefore the treatment goals of the behavioral component of cognitive-behavioral art therapy include (1) helping the client to identify problematic behaviors, (2) assisting the client to learn new behaviors, (3) offering reinforcements and prompts for behaviors, (4) modeling behaviors, (5) offering reality shaping, and (6) helping the client to gain self-control. Behavior modification techniques such as modeling appropriate behavior and operant conditioning are incorporated into the art therapy sessions. A time line in which the client identifies dates and corresponding events works well with the behavioral model enabling clients to identify the temporal connection between events and behaviors. Sticker charts, in which the client is rewarded for appropriate behavior during an art therapy session, have also proven to be beneficial. Visualization and mirroring are both techniques that are elements of the cognitive-behavioral approach. For example, when working with a child who is diagnosed with attention deficit hyperactivity disorder, visualizing and then mirroring the slow and steady behavior of a turtle may be helpful. The child may also be asked to consider that the turtle has a protective shell that keeps it from harm but also modulates its speed. Behaviorists encourage appropriate and desirable behaviors through verbal praise, redirection, and social reinforcements and the therapist helps the client become aware of those situations that cause him or her to present inappropriate or undesired behaviors.

The goals of cognitive-behavioral art therapy are to alter negative thoughts, emotions, and behaviors by addressing cognitive processes and thoughts to produce a change in disturbed thinking. Using a directive approach, the therapist, through identification of negative thoughts and feelings, teaches the client to control his or her cognitive responses in order to eliminate problem symptoms that can lead to emotional disorders such as depression and anxiety. It is believed that the creation of an image of the "negative behavior or anxiety-producing thoughts could be helpful in inducing change" (Malchiodi, 2003, p. 38). An example of the cognitive-behavioral art therapy approach is the work of a teenage client in which film was used as a medium to depict various aspects of conflict resolution.

Developmental Art Therapy

The developmental approach to art therapy "focuses on normal development as the framework for understanding and interviewing with clients whose development is not proceeding according to 'normal' expectations" (Aach-Feldman & Kinkle-Miller, 1987, p. 251). The developmental approach to art therapy can be used with any population. This approach was based largely on the work of Victor Lowenfeld (1947) and expanded on by many art therapists including Anderson (1978, 1992), Henley (1986), Kramer (1971), Silver (1976), and Uhlin (1972).

The developmental approach is rooted in a number of major psychological developmental theories. These theories include, Erickson (1950), Piaget (1954), and of course Lowenfeld (1947). Anderson (1992) summarizes the developmental art therapy approach as having three basic principles: (1) creativity can aid in cognitive and emotional development; (2) there are developmental stages that are evident in a child's art and in a child's behavior with the art materials; and (3) the role of the art therapist must be flexible so that the therapist can at times interact with the client in a directive and action oriented manner and at other times allow for client spontaneity (p. 152).

Developmental art therapists propose that making art stimulates growth and that art can be used as a second language and as a form of communication. According to Anderson (1992), the developmental approach can be used with clients of all ages and is an appropriate treatment approach for individuals who suffer from a wide range of physical and emotional disorders. The developmental art therapy approach is used in clinical and educational settings and can be used in both client assessment and treatment. In educational settings, developmental art therapy techniques can be adapted so that children with a variety of problems and disorders can participate in individual and group art activities alongside their mainstreamed counterparts.

Additional goals in developmental art therapy include increasing client motivation to work on problem behaviors through the use of stimulating material, developing cognitive skills, and enriching and expanding clients' experiences. In the case of a client who suffers from developmental delays or physical disabilities, it may be necessary for the art therapist to adapt the art materials so that he or she can use them effectively and without restriction. For example, the simple adaptation of attaching a sponge to a paint brush may enable a client who has impaired motor skills to create a painting. Similarly, if a piece of sandpaper is placed beneath the art paper on which he or she works, the visually impaired individual can feel exactly what and where he or she is drawing. Such creative adaptations on the part of the art therapist enables all clients to experience the creative art process.

Humanistic Art Therapy

Practitioners of humanistic art therapy believe that the client's own sense of personal well-being is of primary importance and that the emphasis of treatment should be placed on autonomy and personal freedom. According to Malchiodi (2003), the humanistic approach to art therapy developed as a reaction to the psychoanalytic approach that focused on pathology and illness and paid "too much attention to hostility, aggression and neuroses and too little attention to humans' capacity for love, creativity and joy" (p. 58). The humanistic art therapist's role is to work with the client to help him or her develop self-understanding, discover personal meaning, and to create one's own experience. The client plays a central role in this therapy as it is believed that he or she has the ability to find health through art and creativity.

The focus of the humanistic approach to art therapy is on the "acceptance and development of individuals in the present" and upon client wellness and potential for health and growth (Rubin, 1999, p. 162). There are a number of approaches that fall under the humanistic umbrella: client centered or person centered, gestalt, and phenomenological.

Therapists who use the humanistic approach maintain that each client is to be treated and studied as a whole and that the entirety of the person's life is also to be studied and considered (Junge, 1994). Following the outline of Charlotte Buhler (1971), Garai (1987) describes additional goals in humanistic art therapy. These goals include (1) life problem solving, (2) self-actualization, and (3) trust in interpersonal relationships. Humanistic art therapists respect "the person's central role in the therapeutic process" (Malchiodi, 2003, p. 70) and the client's striving to achieve wholeness through integrity, identity, individuation, and idealism.

Humanistic art therapists use a treatment approach that involves helping the client to live a creative life that allows for excitement, self-expression, and intimacy and reinforces the joy of living. The humanistic art therapist takes the stance that clients have "intrapsychic and environmentally caused conflicts" that create mental illnesses (Junge, 1994, p. 144). Therapists who follow this approach believe that most people, in different stages of their lives, struggle to establish stability in their environments, and that such struggles may create problems in their abilities to cope with problems and issues. Humanistic art therapists do not attempt to change or eliminate a client's feeling but seek to help the client in the expression of those feelings. Central to humanistic art therapy is the positive regard of the therapist for clients, their feelings, and also their artwork. The overarching theme in this approach is an optimistic view of human nature and potential. Clients are regarded as being able, with support from the therapist, to shape their own future as they are taught to control their own fate and destiny.

The creation of art within this approach is completely client directed and clients and therapists work with an open studio model. An open studio model is one in which supplies are provided to the client allowing them to master the qualities of various art materials as the art therapist acts as a guide and educator—teaching clients how to use the materials and the possibilities they possess (Spaniol, 2003). All art materials are made available to the client who chooses whatever art medium feels appropriate for his or her personal creativity and self-exploration. This empowerment is what leads to transformation. Activities in humanistic art therapy include dream work visualizations, use of nature, environmental awareness, and affirmations activities. During the client-therapist dialogue, the humanistic art therapist uses open-ended responses which are nonjudgmental and accepting of the client and employs empathetic listening in order to promote client self-understanding and self-acceptance. Many art therapists who use a humanistic approach to art therapy do so because they believe that this approach allows them to provide a supportive client/therapist environment and that through the medium of art clients are freed from the burden of providing "right answers."

Psychoanalytic/Psychodynamic Art Therapy

In the psychoanalytic approach to art therapy, emphasis is placed upon the process of art creation and also upon the subsequent verbalizations made by clients concerning their art work. In this art therapy approach, the client is free to choose his or her own art materials. Lusebrink (1990) describes the psychoanalytic therapy approach as follows, "The Freudian approach is substantiated by the use of symbolic images as an escape from reality; the Jungian interpretation predominates when the images serve a unifying function in regard to the collective past of individual future" (p. 18). Naumberg, who pioneered psychoanalytic art therapy, combined Freudian and Jungian approaches. Naumberg discovered the meaning of her clients' symbols, content, and color usage by questioning and encouraging the client to relate these images to past relationships and experiences.

According to Rosal (1992), the psychoanalytic or psychodynamic approach is best characterized by three main concepts. These concepts are: (1) the creative process taps into the unconscious; (2) art helps to aid in the development of defenses and socially acceptable forms of expression for sexual and aggressive drives or conflicts; and (3) the role of the art therapist is to provide the opportunity for the creative process to take place in a neutral and safe environment (p. 143). The creative process in this approach is the primary focus of the therapy and through the act of creation the client is able to share "difficult unconscious conflicts, wishes, concerns, and drives" (Rosal, 1992, p. 143). The role of the art therapist in the psychoanalytic/psychodynamic approach is not only to encourage client/therapist communication but also to remain neutral, respond to messages in the artwork, understand transference and countertransference, facilitate growth and creative expression, and to use verbal and nonverbal behavior as clues to the client's problems.

Another core theory in the psychoanalytic art therapy model is the issue of self-development. According to Robbins and Sibley (1976) (as reported by Lusebrink, 1990) there are three areas of self development in psychoanalytic/psychodynamic art therapy: (1) building or developing self-image, communication, and interaction with others; (2) revealing and discovering the inner aspects of self; and (3) integrating inner and outer worlds (Lusebrink, 1990, p. 39). Activities or tasks in the psychodynamic art therapy model include the creation of art which explores sexual energy/drive or childhood memories, the creation of symbols of self, symbolic play through puppetry or mask making, and the act of physically destroying a created art piece as a form of sublimation.

Psychoanalytic therapy is based upon the idea that much of our behavior, thoughts, and attitudes are regulated by the unconscious portion of our mind and are not within ordinary conscious control. As the client creates an art piece and then talks about the work he or she has created, the art therapist can assist the client to reveal unconscious or subconscious content revealed by the work and help the client to begin to create order in his or her life.

RESEARCH ON THE EFFECTIVENESS OF ART THERAPY

Art therapy research helps to validate a process that we intuitively know is beneficial. The motivation behind art therapy research "has stemmed from the wish for substantiation of our still young discipline as it takes its place among the more established helping professions" (Wadeson, 1992, p. 1). Art and the creation of art provide a unique source of data. Through the review of client artwork, art therapists can display not only symbols and progress, but also the experiences the therapist has shared with the clients. Art therapy research "paints the picture of the therapeutic process as experienced by the therapist and sometimes by the client" (McNiff, 1998, p. 93). Prinzhorn may have been the first clinician to conduct research on the therapeutic use of art.

Prinzhorn's (1922/1972) documentation *Artistry of the Mentally Ill* analyzed the artwork of mentally ill patients from Austria, Germany, Italy, the Netherlands, and Switzerland. Although he did not explore the history or diagnosis of the patients, he analyzed the images created by them. It is widely believed that because Prinzhorn did not explore the backgrounds of these individuals, his research was actually more objective. "Prinzhorn, like a true scientific researcher, focused on universal conditions such as the tendencies toward order, ornamentation, and repetition that he observed in patient artwork" (McNiff, 1998, p. 99). Prinzhorn's research indicated that individuals with mental illness can use art for a means of self-expression and to help themselves to overcome their limitations.

Much of the research that evaluates the efficacy of art therapy is based on the qualitative methodology of the case study. Case studies describe a "client's history, problem profile, therapeutic plan, and description of the art therapy process" and data is collected through observations, interviews, reviews of records, and the artwork of the client (Rosal, 1989, p. 71). Case studies help clinicians report the art therapy experiences of their clients and enable the therapist to review the entire therapeutic relationship from the initial session through termination. The case study model also allows for the description, discussion, and evaluation of the client's art pieces. Although a case study allows for the in-depth study of one individual, the results are not generalizable to other individuals or other populations and do "not encourage objective evaluations of art therapy" (Rosal, 1989, p. 71). In addition to case studies, methodologies used in art therapy research include, but are not limited to, quasi-experimental designs and assessment research.

Following are descriptions of the two major research methodologies used in art therapy as well as a discussion of scale development and validation.

Case Studies

Mala Betensky conducted research on the relationship between art, making art, and the clients' experiences, communication, self-discovery, and self-expression. Betensky's (1973) research in her book *Self-Discovery Through Self-Expression* describes several case studies complete with drawings and illustrations. Her therapeutic method in working with the clients included asking each client to create an art piece and then discuss the significance of the images produced. As a result of this activity the client was able to make a personal connection to the meaning of their art and a clinical evaluation was made by Betensky. The personal connection of the client to his or her own artwork is what differentiates Betensky's research from that of Prinzhorn who evaluated artwork without any feedback from the client.

Backos and Pagon (1999) used art therapy to aid in inner resolution for adolescent girls suffering from trauma resulting from incest or rape. The adolescent participants ranged in age from 13 to 17 and were receiving therapy through a rape crisis center. The clients were self-referred, referred through Child Protective Services, community agencies, or through the court system. The authors conducted art therapy and support groups for both the adolescents and their parents in which the adolescents met with the therapist for eight weeks and the parents met with the therapist for two weeks. The final session was a group session in which the adolescents, parents, and siblings met together. The group format included rituals for both introduction and closure of each session. Sessions began with the lighting of a candle and ended with the extinction of the candle and the reading of a poem or meditation. Each session commenced with a feeling check called "Myself Tonight." The girls expressed a great deal of anger: anger toward the light sentences received by the perpetrators, anger at themselves (feeling responsible for the assault), and anger related to the loss of their childhood. Many of the girls shared their anxiety over what their futures would hold. As the girls attempted to gain mastery over their feelings of victimization and to become more optimistic about their future, the theme of healing became a focus of the group's dynamics. The group setting and the use of art therapy provided a supportive means for the girls to express their power and to begin the healing process by "offering them ways to become actively involved in changing rigid stereotypical views of rape and incest" and by "provid[ing] an outlet for their anger and outrage" (Backos & Pagon, 1999, p. 131).

Quasi-Experimental Research

Other researchers have used a quasi-experimental approach to evaluate the benefits of art therapy. Quasi-experimental research is similar to experimental research but lacks the random assignment of participants. Banks, Davis, Howard, and McLauglin (1993) studied the effects of directed art activities on the behavior of young children with disabilities. The study was designed to measure the direct effects of art therapy with high risk preschool and primary school students who had disabilities. A multi-element baseline which studies behaviors that can change rapidly and can identify the cause or stimulus for the behaviors was implemented to evaluate various art activities. The results indicated that art activities resulted in the improvement of social behavior with all of the participants. Social behavior includes social skills, social awareness, and social confidence and the ability to use the behaviors appropriately in a situation with others. Social behavior also includes the ability to understand subtle social cues and the feelings of peers. Furthermore, the study suggested that "directed art activities may be effective for improving social behaviors for children" (Banks et al., 1993, p. 239).

Brooke (1995) sought to determine the effectiveness of art therapy in raising the self-esteem of adults who were sexually abused as children. Brooke designed a 20-session art therapy treatment plan that combined both art therapy and group therapy, the goal of which was to increase the ego strength of each individual. Ego strength is the ability to maintain emotional stability, and to handle stress. In a clinical setting ego-strength is said to be a person's capacity to maintain his or her own identity despite psychological pain, distress, turmoil, and conflict between internal forces as well as the demands of reality. Self-esteem, however, is the way a person views him or her self. The six participants of the study were white women between the ages of 20 and 40 years and with an average age of 30. The average age of the control group of five white women was 32 years. The study used the culture free self-esteem inventory for adults (SEI) form AD to measure self-esteem. The results indicated that participants in the experimental group experienced an increase in two of the three self-esteem categories. There was an increase in general self-esteem and social self-esteem but no increase in personal self-esteem. Brooke observed significant themes in the artwork of the participants. For example, many participants displayed guilt and shame in their self-portraits and journals. The art therapy sessions provided a safe environment in which participants were able to share their feelings and their experiences with other women who had undergone similar trauma. The use of art, and an environment based on trust, provided a safe outlet for the women's emotions. Brooke's study presented an alternative therapeutic method of working with this population as well as providing evidence of the quantitative and qualitative changes in self-esteem. "The study provided the members with a coping tool: using art therapy to deal with traumatic situations. The group format served to empower survivors and help them learn appropriate ways to gain control over their lives" (Brooke, 1995, p. 453).

At a hospital in Montreal, Canada, art therapy was used as an intervention to work with patients suffering from somatic complaints and narcissistic identification. Lacroix, Perterson, and Verrier (2001) conducted art therapy research with patients diagnosed with a gastrointestinal disorder called dyspepsia. This disorder, which affects more women than men, includes frequent symptoms of nausea, abdominal pain, and vomiting. According to the authors of the study, 60 percent of women who seek treatment for this disorder have been physically abused and the problems resulting from the abuse are linked to disorders of the gastrointestinal track. The authors of the study maintained that art therapy could be used with patients with somatic symptoms "to give external form or voice to emotions. The patient is encouraged to draw, paint, or sculpt fantasies, dreams, and conflicts after which the patient is invited to extend word associations to the image" (Lacroix et al., 2001, p. 21). The results of the Montreal study indicated that 15 sessions of art therapy gave clients both verbal and visual language. The clients completed the following art experiences during treatment, in addition to others: (1) draw a person, (2) draw your family as food, and (3) draw your frustration. One woman created clay sculptures that represented the dungeon in which she felt trapped by her illness. The final drawing of the treatment sessions was a self-portrait in which she revealed more anxiety, aggressiveness, and assertiveness. The client's ability to express her emotions resulted in an improvement in her symptoms. A follow-up interview months later indicated an even greater reduction in symptoms as well as an increase in her introspection, curiosity, and self-knowledge.

Manning (1987) used art therapy to identify aggression in the drawings of abused children and in her study used the "favorite kind of day" (AFKD) drawing as a monitor of children's emotions. Manning believed that physical abuse is evidenced by the kind of weather the child creates in his or her art work. The directive for the AFKD drawing requires specific weather but enables the child to have "freedom for an individual affectual response" (Manning, 1987, p. 15). The child's freedom in the task enables him or her to reveal much based on the choice of materials and levels of inclement weather. The child is simply asked to draw his or her favorite kind of day. Manning believes that consistently drawn inclement weather may be a sign of abuse. Manning's study consisted of one study group and two control groups. Each group was composed of 10 children between the ages of seven and nine, and was divided in numbers equally between boys and girls. The study or experimental group consisted of children who were abused and were living in a temporary victims of abuse shelter. The first control group consisted of children who were also in a temporary victims of abuse shelter, were from violent homes, but had not been abused. The second control group consisted of children with no known history of abuse. A checklist, which allowed scores that ranged from 3 to 15, indicated that children with a higher checklist score showed the greatest aggression in their drawings. The results indicated that children who experienced abuse and those children from violent homes produced very similar drawings. Both control group participants used outlining as a possible way to create boundaries and rarely included people in their drawings, which may have indicated their need to avoid abusive situations. Results suggested that abused children and those from abusive homes exaggerated the size and movement of inclement weather. Manning suggested that although no one single technique should be used to confirm abuse, higher ratings on the AKFD should warrant concern and further investigation of possible abuse situations.

Art therapy has been implemented with groups to increase locus of control. Rosal (1993) conducted research with 36 children assigned to one of three experimental groups: (1) cognitive-behavioral art therapy, (2) art AS therapy, and (3) control group. Many of the participants, who were in grades four through six, came from families suffering from poverty and instability. In addition to the art therapy approaches, Rosal used three empirical measures to evaluate the outcome of the study: the Children's Nowicki-Strickland Internal-External Locus of Control (CNSIE), the TRS (which monitors children with behavior disorders), and the Personal Construct Drawing Interview (PCDI). The PCDI, which was developed for the study, was used to gauge changes in the participants' attitudes toward school, peers, and people in authoritative positions. Each of the three groups was seen twice a week, for 10 weeks, for 50-minute sessions. Although the quantitative results on the CNSIE and the TRS were not statistically significant, results indicated that "the two art therapy treatment conditions were more effective than a control group in helping the behavior disordered students improve" (Rosal, 1993, p. 236). The results also suggested that art therapy may have helped students with behavior disorders gain self-control and that when discussed the artwork translated emotions and cognition into visual form and reinforced the child's experiences and feelings. Rosal believed that the act of making art mirrored the child's behavior. "A child's movement is reinforced visually by the mark that it produces" (Rosal, 1993, p. 240).

VALIDATION OF ART THERAPY INSTRUMENTS

Mills, Cohen, and Meneses (1993) studied the reliability and validity of the Diagnostic Drawing Series (DDS). The DDS, designed by art therapists, is an art interview in which three drawings are requested from the client. The client is "presented with three pieces of 18 inches by 24 inches white paper and a 12 color box of square, soft chalk pastels" (Mills, Cohen, & Meneses, 1993, p. 83) and asked to draw the following: (1) a picture using the above materials, (2) a tree, and (3) using lines, shapes, and colors, a picture of how the client is feeling. Raters were asked to evaluate the DDS over 23 categories and as some rating criteria allowed for more than two options, each rater made a total of 183 decisions. With over 1,000 cases evaluated for this research, the results indicated that the DDS, which can be utilized with a variety of therapeutic approaches and a variety of populations, is both valid and reliable with 95.7 percent inter-rater reliability.

Neale (1994) investigated the reliability of the Children's Diagnostic Drawing Series (CDDS) to distinguish between children in a treatment group and those in a control group. Neale evaluated 90 subjects from a total of 160. The study findings suggested that participants in the control group were more likely to use "four or more colors in their CDDS than the treatment group" (Neale, 1994, p. 121). Children in the control group were also more likely to use a combination of mixed lines and shapes, whereas those in the treatment group opted for using lines only. Children in the control group were also more likely to include inanimate objects and abstract symbols in their drawing to utilize the entire page to portray an image. Overall findings indicated that the CDDS completed by the children with a diagnosis were different than those children without a diagnosis.

GUIDELINES ON HOW TO USE
ART THERAPY IN PRACTICE

Depending on the setting and the population, as well as the art therapy approach, different guidelines have been developed for the following areas of the therapeutic intervention: environment, assessment/evaluation, materials, and activities which address the goals of treatment.

Environment

Primarily, the physical environment should be structured in such a way that it provides the client and therapist with a safe place in which to interact and create. A secure treatment space will aid the development of trust and confidentiality between client and therapist. The space should be sufficiently supplied with art materials, provide appropriate working surfaces, and have adequate clean-up equipment and storage for art products. Art materials should always be stored in the same area so that the client will be familiar with their location. Materials which are well arranged and consistently available make it easier for the client to create and make choices freely. The room should also be well lit and ventilated and the client should feel that it is "safe" to make a mess in the space as well as having the knowledge that the mess will be easy to clean up. As a demonstration of respect for the client's work and as a means of enhancing the therapeutic relationship, the therapist must provide sufficient and secure storage space for the client's artwork.

Assessment/Evaluation

In order to determine the appropriate form of treatment it is essential that the art therapist conduct an assessment or evaluation of the client. As in all therapeutic relationships, mutual respect is crucial. Client and therapist together must clarify the contractual expectations of the therapeutic relationship to include issues of confidentiality, fees (in private practice situations), scheduling of appointments, and duration of therapy. If the art therapist is part of a treatment team, he or she must discuss the client's needs with the other team members so that treatment issues, scheduling of additional therapies, and open communication among the clinicians is ensured.

As a means of client assessment, it is usual, during the first session of art therapy treatment for a series of drawings to be collected from the client. Three of the most frequently collected drawings in the initial session are the House-Tree-Person (HTP), the Kinetic Family Drawing (KFD), and the Draw-A-Person (DAP) test. The HTP, developed by Buck (1948), indicates how clients feel about themselves in the present, past, and the current world in which they live. Rubin states that the HTP has proved to be "most fruitful as a source of client's self-discovery" (Rubin, 1987, p. 156). Using a number two graphite pencil, and a separate piece of white paper for each drawing clients are instructed to draw a house, tree, and a person. This assessment is typically completed on a sheet of 7" × 8.5" paper although 8.5" × 11" paper is often substituted. Because of their familiarity to most clients, the house, tree, and person are selected as subjects for clients' drawings. Many art therapists do not use the HTP as an assessment, but rather as a device to become more familiar with the symbolic content, the line quality of the client's work, and the emotional state of the client. The KFD, developed by Burns and Kaufman (1970), requires that the client draw a picture of his or her family engaged in an activity. By means of this image the therapist is able to ascertain family dynamics and interactions and how the client perceives his or her family. The KFD should only be used when the client has developed a sense of trust and mutual respect in the therapeutic relationship and therefore is most suitable for use in individual therapy sessions and for later stages of group therapy. Using the DAP technique developed by Ogden (1977), the therapist asks the client to draw a whole person of the same gender as him or her self and then another drawing of a person of the opposite gender. The persons created by the client help the therapist to identify any difficulties in concepts the client may have in relationships with people of the same or opposite gender. Often emotional distress is related to a poor self-image and so the art therapist also considers the size and placement of the figure to determine the client's levels of self-concept and self-esteem. According to Lusebrink (1990), the problem of self-image can "contribute to increased experienced stress and ultimately to a disease. Developmentally, the body image precedes the self-image as a representation of self" (p. 235). Although all of the previously described assessments are commonly used by art therapists, little empirical research has been conducted to validate the use of these instruments as accurate assessment tools (Kaplan, 2003).

Materials

Art materials are an essential part of art therapy practice and although it is not necessary for art therapists to be artists, they must be familiar with various art materials and the specific properties of those materials. The therapist's familiarity with art materials will enable him or her to provide technical assistance to clients when necessary. In addition to the appropriate tools needed for clients to draw, tools for painting, modeling, and constructing a full array of two-dimensional and three-dimensional objects should be available. Art supplies should include, but are not limited to:

1. Paper in a variety of sizes, colors, and textures in addition to other surfaces on which clients can draw or paint.
2. A range of drawing materials including paints (acrylic, tempera, oil, and watercolor), markers (both fine and broad felt tipped), pastels (chalk and oil), graphite pencils, colored pencils, erasers, palettes for use in paint mixing.
3. Various kinds of clay including air drying clay, plastecine, and earth clay. A kiln will be necessary for firing earth clay and glazed earth clay pieces.
4. An assortment of collage materials such as magazines, colored construction paper, glitter, sequins, string, yarn, found objects, bits of cloth.
5. Art room staples such as white glue, tape, staplers, scissors, containers for water, brushes.

All art materials for children who are 12 years of age and younger and for those with developmental disabilities should be certified by the Arts and Crafts Materials Institute as AP or CP nontoxic. Art supplies can be purchased from office supply stores, art supply stores, teacher supply stores, and discount stores such as Wal-Mart, Kmart, or Target.

Each art medium is characterized by its own specific properties and is considered to be either fluid or resistive in nature. The following section of the chapter focuses on a description of the various art media used in art therapy.

Chalk Pastels

Chalk pastels are offered in a variety of colors and can be used with both their broad or narrow edges to provide either large coverage of areas or fine details. This media is considered fairly fluid and difficult to control as the pastels create dust, which can be messy and may result in unwanted fingerprints.

Oil Pastels

Oil pastels are available in a variety of colors and sizes and the texture of the pastels provides for blending of colors. Color can be applied by using either the side or the tip of the pastel and coverage of the paper varies from light to dense depending on the pressure utilized by the client. This medium can be difficult for clients to control and is considered to be relatively fluid.

Clay (Earth)

Earth clay is moldable and controllable enabling the client to squeeze the material, and thus release tension. Other clay techniques, such as wedging, modeling, and stretching, provide additional ways to release anger. This medium offers a tactile experience and is considered to be fairly resistive when used in its dry form, but very fluid when combined with water.

Clay (Plastecine)

Plastecine is a hard oily clay and is very resistive. It comes in many colors and is nondrying. Although it is reusable, the therapist should be aware that the material is likely to hold germs and there is a possibility of germ transference between clients.

Finger Paints

Finger paints are the most fluid of all media. Finger paints come in a variety of colors and are often used on both finger paint paper (which has a glossy surface) and drawing paper (which is more absorbent). The use of fingers rather than a brush in creating a painting results in immediate regression for the client and the creative process can become very messy.

Paint—Tempera

Tempera paint is a medium commonly used in classrooms and in art therapy because it is very inexpensive. This paint is very fluid, comes in a variety of colors and its consistency makes it easy to mix and create new colors although application of too many layers of paint will result in cracking of the artwork. The fluidity of tempera paint can cause clients to regress and when applied in broad strokes may have a calming effect.

Paint—Acrylic

Acrylic paint is more expensive than tempera but is a more professional grade of art material. Acrylic paint is simple to mix, dilutes well with water, dries quickly, and is easy to clean up. This media is considered to be moderately fluid.

Paint—Watercolor

Because of its fluidity, watercolor paint is considered to be the most difficult medium for clients to master and strokes or marks once executed cannot be changed as they are difficult to conceal. Completed watercolor paintings are characterized by a transparent quality.

Materials for the Creation of Collage

In order to create a collage, the client uses fabric, paper, magazines, and found objects to produce two-dimensional and three-dimensional images. Hence, a ready supply of textured materials and fabrics of all types as well as different kinds of adhesives should be available for clients who wish to work in this medium. Clients often add drawn and painted images to their collages and hence all other types of aforementioned art media also should be accessible to the client. Because the creation of a collage involves the client in many tactile activities (ripping, tearing, cutting, gluing, and manipulation of various materials) it is considered to be a very resistive medium.

Art materials should be well organized with appropriate and accessible storage spaces. The art therapist needs to be flexible in the use of art materials, and art therapy space may need to be adapted to meet the client's needs. Such adaptations may include lowering or raising of tables and chairs, providing or creating broad-handled instruments for someone with poor fine motor skills, removing distractions from the client's working-space, or reducing or limiting the number of art materials available to the client. According to Rubin (1984), it is important that the art materials are developmentally appropriate for the client's "developmental level, degree of coordination, previous experiences, particular interests, and special needs" (p. 31). With the appropriate structure, materials, environment, and therapeutic modality, the client "may discover their own unique tastes and preferences, their own favorite forms of expression" (Rubin, 1984, p. 32).

Art Therapy Activities

A major role of all art therapists is to create interventions and art activities based on the needs, interests, media preferences, and goals of each individual client. The following is a sampling of art therapy activities commonly used in practice.

Scribble Chase

Scribble chase is an activity that is often used as an icebreaker for a new group of clients. The materials used are markers, butcher paper, and 18" × 24" paper. Smaller sizes of paper can be utilized when the larger-size paper appears to overwhelm the clients. The procedure for the activity is as follows:

1. Clients select a partner.
2. Each client chooses a different colored marker.
3. Clients decide which person will be the leader and which will be the follower.
4. Leader begins to scribble randomly and the partner follows the leader's scribble.
5. Clients are informed that they may switch roles midway through the scribble exercise.
6. Clients are asked to identify five images from the scribble and to label them.
7. Clients are instructed to get into groups of four. The group of four is then asked to identify and agree upon five images selected from the work of the two sets of partners.

8. Clients are instructed to form a larger group of eight and again choose only five images. In smaller group settings this step may be unnecessary.
9. The group is then instructed to create a story about the five images and using the images selected, place the story onto butcher block paper. Each group shares its stories and images with the larger group and group members discuss how they feel about the experience.

For the participants in the scribble chase, the exercise may serve as a good kinesthetic release and this activity helps both the clients and the therapist to identify group leaders and how well individuals cooperate and interact with one another. It also reveals to the therapist which clients feel anxious about sharing their art space with others. An added benefit of the scribble exercise is that clients are required to compromise with each other at many points throughout the activity. Cognitive responses to the activity include the observation of images, problem solving, and communication. Personal symbols and group symbols may represent the personal and group experience and enable individuals to find a common ground which then evolves into the group image and story.

Media Properties

Media properties is an activity that helps the therapist to understand the needs, comfort level, and skills of the client in relation to various art media. Materials for this activity include tempera paint, finger paints, clay, plasticene, oil pastels, chalk pastels, watercolor, collage materials, 18" × 24" paper, and paint brushes. Tables are arranged with different art materials and the client rotates between the different tables creating art pieces or simply experiencing each medium. The client rates each medium for its usability. This activity exposes the client to the various art media that will be available to him or her throughout the course of therapy.

Body Tracing (Ideal Self)

Body tracing is an individual or group activity that helps the client to become aware of body image and problems related to that image. Materials needed for this activity include butcher-block paper and various drawing and painting materials such as tempera paints, oil pastels, chalk pastels, and collage materials such as fabric pieces, found objects (objects found such as buttons, paper, labels, flowers, leaves, twigs, bottle caps, etc.), and glitter. Each client is asked to select a partner (usually of the same gender) and partners trace each other's bodies onto butcher-block paper. The body tracing can also be implemented in an individual session with the therapist as the tracer. The client is instructed to decorate his or her own tracing in order to create an image of the ideal self. The client is also encouraged to draw inside and outside of the body outline with the result that each participant is able to see him or her self in a concrete way. Each client processes his or her discoveries and reactions to his or her own body depiction with the group and also shares observations concerning the work of other group members. Although this activity can be both empowering and beneficial for the client, it may be especially threatening and traumatic for those who have experienced trauma/sexual abuse, or have severe body image issues. The therapist must also be aware that the display of the body tracing before other clients may make the client feel vulnerable and exposed. Body tracing should be conducted only when the individual client, the group, and the therapist have built a strong mutual therapeutic relationship.

Family of Origin

The family of origin activity incorporates both art-making and role-playing. The client is asked to create his or her family of origin from plastecine and to place the family on a tray. The client is instructed to role-play the family's dynamics, acting out the perceived role of each individual in the family. The client is then instructed to reposition the family members, as he or she would like them to be and encouraged to discuss how he or she feels about the new family grouping. The use of the family of origin activity provides the client with the opportunity to achieve reflective distance and allows him or her to identify family issues, roles and dynamics, and what coping skills are used within the family. With a well-established group, group members may take the role of various family members while the client represents him or her self thus enabling him or her to gain insight into issues within the family and the rules by which the family operates. The group can then aid the client to process both the art-making and role-playing experiences. It is essential that this activity be implemented only when the group has bonded and there exists a strong sense of mutual trust between group members.

CASE STUDY

Bobby was a six-year-old Bahamian male diagnosed with cerebral palsy. He was born in a government run medical hospital in Nassau, Bahamas, and because of his physical problems, had been abandoned by his mother immediately after his birth. There were no family members or guardians listed for Bobby and he had lived his entire life in the hospital.

Bobby was very small in stature and weighed approximately 25 pounds. He appeared clean, was clothed, and was fed daily by the hospital staff. Reports indicated that Bobby had occasional interaction with hospital staff and had undergone some unspecified therapy at the hospital. A two-week study abroad program run by a university in the southern United States, introduced art therapy briefly to the local community center for the physically disabled in Nassau. Four graduate level art therapy students, one graduate level drama therapy student, one recent art therapy graduate, and one art therapy professor developed and implemented developmental adaptive art therapy for approximately 20 children (3-11 years old) with various disabilities. Developmental adaptive art therapy is based on the concept of normalization, providing opportunities for the client to lead a "normal" life. It is a form of art therapy that provides that "all art therapy experiences can be adapted to meet the unique [developmental and physical] needs of the disabled child" (Anderson, 1992, p. 162). According to Anderson, there are four categories of adaptation:

1. adaptation of physical environment
2. adaptation of the art tools and media
3. adaptation of the instructional sequence
4. technological adaptations

Accompanied by a nurse, Bobby was brought to the center every day to participate in the program. As Bobby had not previously participated in any activities at the center, the staff was unfamiliar with his strengths, weaknesses, or general ability levels. The nurse who accompanied Bobby informed the art therapists and the staff that Bobby was unable to do anything and would only be able to watch the other children. She stated that he was unable to walk, talk, or move his arms. When moved into one of the group rooms in a stroller with little back support, he sat in a slumped position with his arms and legs drawn in toward his torso and his head turned to one side. Immediately the art therapist and art therapy students decided to use an adaptive art therapy approach in their work with Bobby. The basic principles of art therapy dictate that if the focus of the therapy is to enable the client to participate in normalizing experiences, the art materials, the room, and the activities are to be adaptive to meet the needs of that client (Anderson, 1992). Bobby's severe physical limitations necessitated that the therapists make many adaptations to the art materials he was to use. The therapists taped a piece of paper to the side and wheeled Bobby over to it thus enabling him to draw. He was then given a selection of large crayons. Although nonverbal, Bobby made his crayon color choice clear by picking up the crayon with his feet and beginning to draw. By dropping the crayon he was using and holding his toes open until the correct color was placed between them he was able to signal to the therapist working with him that he wanted another color. Even though not representational, Bobby's drawings appeared to be controlled scribbles.

Bobby quickly developed a rapport with the art therapist. He was not verbally communicative but he began to smile and attempt to turn his head to find the art therapist. The art therapist decided to take Bobby out of the stroller and place him on the floor on her lap thus providing him with more support and freedom of movement and positioning him at the same eye level as herself. Once on the floor, Bobby worked very hard at turning his head to view his artwork. Gradually, the art therapist gave Bobby more difficult tasks to complete and he was able to follow directions with multiple components. It seemed clear that Bobby's cognitive skills were age appropriate and he was able to concentrate on art projects for well over two hours at a time before becoming distracted. Bobby completed all of the scheduled art activities designed by the art therapist, including drawing, painting a mural, making puppets out of paper bags and felt, and constructing a papier-mache animal. All of the art activities selected by the therapist were based on the book *Giraffes Can't Dance* by Giles Andreae and Guy Parker-Rees (1999). This children's book was chosen because it conveys a positive message about being different.

During the last few days of the art therapy program, Bobby seemed to thrive. He appeared very proud of his paper-mache alligator and especially enjoyed times when the staff used it to interact between Bobby and themselves. At the closing ceremony of the study abroad program, the minister of social services and community development, who had spearheaded the university/community center joint program, spoke about the tremendous strides made by Bobby. Bobby was very pleased, smiled broadly, and using his feet, clapped for himself. Bobby's responses during the two-week program and his reaction to the minister's speech indicated that Bobby's cognitive skills were intact and that his disability was limited to his physical condition. Bobby had been attempting to verbally communicate throughout the two-week program, but he only made soft sounds which were indecipherable to the therapists and staff. On the last day of the program however, as they sat together, he clearly said the therapist's name. Bobby's tremendous progress during such a short program encouraged the staff at the community center and at his residential hospital to provide him with additional stimulation and to continue to use art as a way to facilitate his communication skills, improve his fine and gross motor skills, and to increase his self-esteem.

CONTRAINDICATIONS FOR ART THERAPY?

With the ability to help so many people, are there contraindications for the use of art therapy? Adaptations of the art therapy tasks, materials, sequence, or environment can be adjusted for most situations and populations. There are, however, situations, client history, and conditions in which art therapy must be used with caution.

Untrained Clinicians

First and foremost, art therapy treatment and interventions should only be utilized by a trained art therapist. Utilizing art therapy techniques and processes without proper training and supervision may lead to the unveiling of thoughts and emotions that the untrained clinician is not aware of or may be unable to resolve, thus leading the client to greater states of anxiety or depression. Therefore, the use of art therapy is contraindicated for untrained professionals with any and all populations, that is not to say that clinicians in other fields cannot use art as a therapeutic tool, it is only to say that attempting techniques indicated here may cause harm when used inappropriately. Art has been used in many forms of therapy and we must all be aware of the power of the process and the symbols clients create as well as the magnitude of the discoveries inherent in the process.

Cautious Use of Art Therapy with Certain Populations

Art therapists working with clients with schizophrenia or disso- ciative disorder should be thoughtful of their choice of art therapy ac- tivities. The use of guided imagery and fantasy-based art therapy activities are to be used with great care (if at all), as the client's reality testing may already be impaired. "The art therapy technique of scrib- bling, abstraction or any fantasy-delusional, spontaneous artwork should be avoided" (Crespo, 2003, p. 191). According to Crespo, the art therapist must also address the use of certain art materials as the stimulus of the medium may encourage regression or fantasy. Art therapy should also be used with caution when attempting to address topics such as empathy, boundaries, and reality testing. Structured activities that are based in reality can foster insight, help with problem solving skills, and encourage grounding.

Clients with self injurious behavior (intentional and repeated burn- ing, cutting, scratching, or bruising oneself) can often benefit from art therapy as it can help to promote healing, communication, and comfort. Many of the tools used in art making, however, may be used by the client to injure him or her self. Again, great care must be used when deciding on appropriate art medium and interventions with this population. Activities that create a loss of control, failure, or a nega- tive outcome can trigger the cycle of self-injurious behavior.

It is unadvisable to use certain techniques with clients with eating disorders or a history of sexual abuse. An art therapy task such as a body tracing (in which the client's body is traced by the therapist or a group member) can cause adverse reactions and trigger memories of past abuse or current poor body image thoughts and poor self-esteem and send the client spiraling into lower states of depression or self-injurious behaviors. These issues are addressed in the education, training, and supervision of pre-service art therapists so that such inappropriate tasks are not given or are given under the watchful eye of a supervisor.

CONCLUSION

Art therapy is a unique tool that aids in health and healing. The combination of art and psychology within the art therapy approach provides clients with an alternative form of therapeutic communication and self-expression. In their work with clients, therapists may use one or more of the several approaches which fall within the discipline of art therapy but the underlying goal of each art therapy stance is to provide a safe vehicle in which clients who may otherwise be inarticulate are enabled through their artwork to express their experiences, fears, wishes, and hopes. "Patients can, and often do, with the help of a trained art therapist draw their way back to health" (Drachnik, 1995, p. 68).

A tenet of art therapy is the belief that "drawings tend to tell more about the artist who created them than about the objects portrayed" (Drachnik, 1995, p. vi). It is this principle that makes the art therapy approach suitable for clients of all ages and abilities for the art therapist does not seek to judge the client's artwork but allows the work itself to speak on the client's behalf.

REFERENCES

Aach-Feldman, S. & Kunkle-Miller, C. (1987). A developmental approach to art therapy. In J.A. Rubin (Ed.), *Approaches to art therapy: Theory and technique* (pp. 251-274). Levittown, PA: Brunner/Mazel, Inc.

American Art Therapy Association. (2005). Retrieved January 11, 2005, from www.arttherapy.org.

American Heritage Dictionary of the English Language (4th ed.). (2000). Boston: Houghton Mifflin Company.

Anderson, F.E. (Ed.). (1992). *Art for all the children*. Springfield, IL: Charles C Thomas.

Andreae, G. & Parker-Rees, G. (1999). *Giraffes can't dance.* New York: Orchard Books.

Art Therapy: About the program. www.drexel.edu/cnhp/art-therapy/about.csp.

Backos, A.K. & Pagon, B.E. (1999). Finding a voice: Art therapy with female adolescents sexual abuse survivors. *Art Therapy: Journal of the American Art Therapy Association, 16*(3), 126-132.

Banks, S., Davis, P., Howard, V., & McLaughlin, T.F. (1993). The effects of directed art activities on the behavior of young children with disabilities: A multi-element baseline analysis. *Art Therapy: Journal of the American Art Therapy Association, 10*(4), 235-240.

Betensky, M. (1973). *Self-discovery through self-expression: Use of art in psychotherapy with children and adolescents.* Springfield, IL: Charles C Thomas.

Brooke, S. (1995). Art therapy with sexual abuse survivors. *The Arts in Psychotherapy, 22* (5), 447-466.

Buck, J.N. (1948). The H-T-P technique: A qualitative and quantitative scoring manual. *Journal of Clinical Psychology, 10,* 317-396.

Buhler, C. (1971). Basic theoretical concepts of humanistic psychology. *American Psychologists, 24,* 378-386.

Burns, R.C. & Kaufman, S.H. (1970). *Kinetic family drawings (KFD).* New York: Brunner/Mazel, Inc.

Crespo, V.R. (2003). Art therapy as an approach for working with schizophrenic patients. *International Journal of Psychotherapy, 8*(3), 183-193.

Dalley, T. (1984). *Art as therapy: An introduction to the use of art as a therapeutic technique.* London: Tavistock/Routledge.

Dalley, T., Case, C., Schaverien, J., Weir, F., Halliday, D., Hall, P.N., & Waller, D. (1987). *Images of art therapy: New developments in theory and practice.* London: Tavistock/Routledge.

Drachnik, C. (1995). *Interpreting metaphors in children's drawings.* Burlingame, California: Abbeygate Press.

Erickson, E. (1950). *Childhood and society.* New York: Norton.

Gantt, L. & Schmal, M. (1974). *Art therapy: A bibliography,* January 1940-June 1973. Rockville, MD: National Institute of Mental Health, DHEW Publication No. (Adm) 74-81.

Garai, J.E. (1987). A humanistic approach to art therapy. In J.A. Rubin (Ed.), *Approaches to art therapy: Theory and technique* (pp. 188-207). Levittown, PA: Brunner/Mazel, Inc.

Henley, D.K. (1986). Approaching artistic sublimation in low-functioning individuals. *Art Therapy, 3*(2), 115-124.

Jones, D. (1983). An art therapist personal record. *Art Therapy: Journal of the American Art Therapy Association, 1,* 22-25.

Junge, M.B. (1994). *A history of art therapy in the United States.* Mundelein, IL: American Art Therapy Association.

Kagin, S.L. & Lusebrink, V.B. (1978) The expressive therapies continuum. *Art Psychotherapy, 5*(4), 171-179.

Kaplan, F.E. (2003). Art-based assessments. In C.A. Malchiodi (Ed.), *Handbook of art therapy* (pp. 25-35). New York: The Guilford Press.

Knapp, N.M. (1992). Tabulated review of diagnostic use of art as preliminary resource for research with alzheimers disease. *American Journal of Art Therapy, 31*(2), 46-63. Retrieved November 17, 2005, from www.ephost@epnet.com.

Kramer, E. (1958). *Art therapy in a children's community.* Springfield, IL: Charles C Thomas.

Kramer, E. (1971). *Art as therapy with children.* New York: Schocken Books.

Kwiatkowska, H. (1962). Family art therapy: Experiments with a new technique. *Bulletin of Art Therapy, 1,* 3-15.

Lacroix, L., Peterson, L., & Verrier, P. (2001). Art therapy, somatization, and narcissistic identification. *Art Therapy: Journal of the American Art Therapy Association, 18*(1), 20-26.

Landgarten, H. (1981). *Clinical art therapy: A comprehensive guide.* New York: Brunner/Mazel.

Lark, C. (2001). *Art therapy overview: An informal background paper.* www.arttherapy.com/arttherapyoverview.htm.

Levick, M.F. (1967). The goals of the art therapist as compared to those of the art teacher. *Journal of Albert Einstein Medical Center, 15,* 157-170.

Lowenfeld, V. (1947). *Creative and mental growth* (3rd ed.). New York: Macmillan.

Lusebrink, V.B. (1990). *Imagery and visual expression in therapy.* New York: Plenum Press.

Malchiodi, C.A. (1998). *The art therapy sourcebook.* Los Angels: Lowell House.

Malchiodi, C.A. (Ed.). (2003). *Handbook of art therapy.* New York: The Guilford Press.

Malchiodi, C.A. (2003). Humanistic approaches. In C.A. Malchiodi (Ed.), *Handbook of art therapy* (pp. 58-71). New York: The Guilford Press.

Manning, T.M. (1987). Aggression depicted in abused children's drawings. *The Arts in Psychotherapy, 14,* 15-24.

McNiff, S. (1998). *Art-based research.* London: Jessica Kingsley Publishers.

Mills, A., Cohen, B., & Meneses, J.Z. (1993). Reliability and validity tests of the diagnostic drawing series. *The Arts in Psychotherapy, 20,* 83-88.

Naumberg, M. (1966). *Dynamically oriented art therapy: Its principles and practice.* Chicago: Magnolia Street Publishers.

Neale, E.L. (1994). The children's diagnostic drawing series. *Art Therapy: Journal of the American Art Therapy Association, 11*(2), 119-126.

Ogden, D.P. (1977). *Psychodiagnostics and personality assessments: A handbook* (2nd ed.). Los Angeles: Western Psychological Services.

Piaget, J. (1954). *The construction of reality in the child.* New York: Basic Books.

Prinzhorn, H. (1922/1972). *Artistry of the mentally ill.* New York: Springer-Verlag. (Original English translation published in 1922.)

Rhyne, J. (1973). *The gestalt art experience.* Monterey, CA: Brooks/Cole.

Rosal, M.L. (1989). Master's papers in art therapy: Narrative or research case studies? *The Arts in Psychotherapy, 16,* 71-75.

Rosal, M.L. (1992). Approaches to art therapy with children. In F.E. Anderson (Ed.), *Art for all the children: Approaches to art therapy for children with disabilities.* Springfield, IL: Charles C Thomas.

Rosal, M.L. (1993). Comparative group art therapy research to evaluate changes in locus of control in behavior disordered children. *The Arts in Psychotherapy, 20,* 231-241.

Rowe, F.B., Crews, W.D., & Finger, F.W. (1993). John N. Buck (1906-1983): Did he practically establish clinical psychology in Virginia? *Journal of Clinical Psychology, 49*(3), 428-434.

Rubin, J.A. (1978). *Child art therapy: Understanding and helping children grow through art.* Sydney, Australia: Van Nostrand Reinhold.

Rubin, J.A. (1984). *The art of art therapy.* New York: Brunner/Mazel, Inc.

Rubin, J.A. (Ed.). (1987). *Approaches to art therapy: Theory and technique.* Levittown, PA: Brunner/Mazel, Inc.

Rubin, J.A. (1999). *Art therapy: An introduction.* Philadelphia, PA: Brunner/Mazel.

Silver, R. (1976). Using art to evaluate and develop cognitive skills. *American Journal of Art Therapy, 16,* 11-19.

Silver, R. (1987). A cognitive approach to art therapy (pp. 233-250). In J.A. Rubin (Ed.), *Approaches to art therapy: Theory and practice.* Levittown, PA: Brunner/ Mazel. Incorporated.

Spaniol, S. (2003). Art therapy with adults with severe mental illness. In C.A. Malchiodi (Ed.), *Handbook of art therapy* (pp. 268-280). New York: Guilford Press.

Uhlin, D.M. (1972). *Art for exceptional children.* Dubuque, IA: William C. Brown Company.

Ulman, E. (1975). Art therapy: Problems of definition. In E. Ulman & P. Dachinger (Eds.), *Art therapy in theory and practice.* New York: Schoken.

Wadeson, H. (1980). *Art psychotherapy.* New York: John Wiley and Sons, Inc.

Wadeson, H., Durkin, J., & Perach, D (Eds.). (1989). *Advances in art therapy.* New York: John Wiley.

Chapter 6

Psychodrama

Trudy K. Duffy

INTRODUCTION

Psychodrama is a type of therapeutic theater developed by J. L. Moreno. It is collaborative, improvisational theater with great adaptability to treatment, education, and community settings. Moreno (1943, 1985) described its milieu "as broad as the wings of imagination can make it, yet inclusive of every particle of our real worlds" (p. 328). In psychodrama, people bring their life experiences to the stage. They do not simply talk about their concerns; they act out the situations and relationships that give rise to such concerns. They gain insight from the action itself. On the psychodrama stage, participants explore personal and social situations, gain new perspective, heal from hurt and neglect, learn life skills, and practice new behavior.

HISTORY OF PSYCHODRAMA

Origin

Psychodrama was developed by Jacob Levy Moreno (1889-1974). Born in Bucharest, Moreno was raised and educated in Vienna, an environment of great intellectual and political ferment that promoted his inventiveness. Moreno obtained his medical degree in 1917 and

Introduction to Alternative and Complementary Therapies
© 2008 by The Haworth Press, Taylor & Francis Group. All rights reserved.
doi:10.1300/5987_06

practiced as a physician; he also became known as a scientist, social activist, writer, poet, director of improvisational theater, and editor of a literary journal (Marineau, 1989).

Moreno's idea for psychodrama came from observing children's play in Vienna's Ausgarten, a place he often visited as a young medical student. Moreno noted how children took on roles of parents and other significant people and things in their lives and how they seemed to gain a sense of control and satisfaction from playing out familiar scenes. He discovered a similar effect with adults when he created his spontaneity theater, a theater in which people in the audience suggested topics from the newspaper and then with the aid of a few trained actors improvised short dramas. Eventually, Moreno brought theater techniques to his psychiatric practice; his patients experienced less mental distress and greater readiness for social interaction.

Moreno recognized the importance of small groups, both as social networks and as microcosms of society. He noted the therapeutic benefits of member-to-member interaction and called this "group psychotherapy" (1932, 1957). He said, "Every individual is a therapeutic agent of the other individual, and every group is a therapeutic agent of every other group" (Moreno, 1957, p. xii). He believed that the "whole of mankind" must be the focus of any truly therapeutic procedure (Moreno, 1968). These ideas had roots in Moreno's work as a community physician. For example, when providing medical services to prostitutes in Vienna, he recognized the impact of social and political policies. He invited the women to come together, similar to a support group, to have coffee and talk about their lives, also to advocate for civil treatment from the police and better medical services. Moreno's broad approach contrasted sharply with Freud's highly individualized psychoanalysis (Moreno, 1943) as the following popular story illustrates. Dr. Moreno is said to have conversed briefly with Dr. Freud in Vienna following one of Freud's lectures on dreams. "And what do you do?" Freud asked. Moreno replied, "Well, Dr. Freud, I start where you leave off. You meet people in the artificial setting of your office; I meet them on the street and in their homes. You analyze their dreams; I give them the courage to dream again" (Rowan, personal communication, 1971).

Psychodrama in the United States

In 1925, Moreno immigrated to New York, where he continued to practice psychiatry and develop his ideas. He worked at the Training School for Girls in Hudson and was director of research under the New York State Social Welfare Department. He directed a theater in New York City much like the spontaneity theatre in Vienna (Moreno, 1947, 1983). He opened a sanatorium in Beacon, New York, and built a psychodrama stage for patient treatment (later used for psychodrama training). His notes from Beacon demonstrate careful and comprehensive work with patients having problems with depression, anxiety, psychosis, dementia, and alcoholism. At a period prior to antipschotic medications, Moreno dared to take patients onto the psychodrama stage and into their hallucinations, with staff serving as auxiliaries. He found that, over time, patients became less attached to the exact details of their delusions and allowed greater flexibility in the script. Ultimately, patients gained confidence in their ability to move from hallucinations back into reality, giving them increased tolerance and control. Moreno's treatment in all cases involved family members and others from patients' social networks.

Moreno initiated the American Society of Group Psychotherapy and Psychodrama in 1942, the International Congress of Group Psychotherapy in 1951, which is now the International Association of Group Psychotherapy, and created avenues for education through journals of sociology and psychodrama.

A significant addition to the development of psychodrama came in the person of Zerka Toeman, Moreno's wife, collaborator and coauthor. Complementing his focus on broad social issues, Zerka Moreno introduced a personal, interior use of psychodrama that has come to be known as classical psychodrama. Zerka Moreno continues today to be a significant teacher and mentor to individuals and organizations of psychodrama throughout the world.

THEORY OF PSYCHODRAMA

Psychodrama theory reflects the grandness of Moreno's thought. He envisioned creation as ongoing and people as having the strength and responsibility to be cocreators and healers of the world, along with the ultimate maker, Godhead (Moreno, 1946, 1985). His core concepts regarding spontaneity and creativity, social choices and the interdependence of individuals and society, and the links between mind and body are presented in greatly simplified form below.

Principles of Spontaneity and Creativity

The word *spontaneity* comes from Latin *sua sponte,* meaning "of free will" or "moving by itself"; it suggests a readiness to create, to think afresh (Blatner, 2000). *Creativity* is action sparked by spontaneity that results in a product of some sort—a strategy, book, invention, instrument, law, environment, and so on. Products get conserved as part of cultures, providing some stability. These conserves become stale and irrelevant, however, spontaneity must be activated again to assure the vitality and health of individuals and society.

Despite its importance in the cycle described above, spontaneity is not a well-developed aptitude in humans. Moreno said that individuals with spontaneity can respond to old situations in a new ways; they can respond to new situations competently (Moreno, 1946, 1985). Spontaneous responses, by his definition, are novel, appropriate, and effective, not impulsive or irresponsible. Spontaneity cannot be stored, so it has to be produced to meet the demand of each situation. Anxiety and physiological changes resulting from trauma can decrease a person's capacity for being spontaneous and creative. Fortunately, training and practice can develop this capacity.

Psychodrama demands, teaches, and trains spontaneity by placing participants in situations that require novel responses. Over and over again, role-players in psychodrama are asked to call upon their creativity in order to provide the deep and complicated responses necessary to fulfill their roles in action. Psychodrama trains people to think on their feet. It encourages risk-taking and allows a large enough margin for failure, or what may feel like failure, so that participants learn to move through situations that may have previously baffled them, shut them down, or rendered them silent. It allows them to experiment with new behaviors, alternate responses, and explore fresh points of view (Dayton, 1994).

Social Choices and Connections

Moreno conducted extensive scientific studies of the choices people made in social relationships. He developed a measurement system (sociometry) that quantifies social connections and identifies subgroups, leaders, and isolates. His findings contribute to small group and sociological theories. Some basic ideas are the following: society is made up of individuals and their essential social relationships, called *social atoms*. The well-being of individuals is related to the adequacy of their social atoms. When people meet, they rely on a reciprocal flow of feeling between them, called *tele;* this is a kind of correspondence that takes place instantly and affects social choices. Interpersonal learning occurs through authentic encounters between persons in which each momentarily views the world through the other's eyes (Moreno, 1934, 1953).

Health and Healing

Moreno was clear that mind and body are connected and that experiences are encoded in both. Therefore, treatment has to include both. "No moment can be bypassed because every moment is in the being and no part can be left out because every part is in the being" (Moreno & Moreno, 1975, p. 212). Treatment on the psychodrama stage is successful because it condenses a person's situation to its essential "parts" and brings the "moments" to the present, so they can be experienced as if for the first time. In psychodrama, action is primary. Putting it developmentally, Zerka Moreno said, "Action precedes speech. Speech is a later development and is not the royal route to the psyche" (Holmes, Karp, & Watson, 1994, p. xii).

J. L. and Zerka Moreno were forerunners to current methods of treating trauma. Today, there is substantial evidence that trauma gets set in the sensorimotor part of the brain and cannot be easily translated into the symbolic language used by traditional therapies (van der Kolk & van der Hart, 1995). Action methods, such as psychodrama, can access these memories and assist in the processing and integration of the trauma. In addition, psychodrama can assist in retraining. "Once the traumatic experiences have been located in time and place, a person can start making distinctions between current life stresses and past trauma and decrease the impact of the trauma on present experience" (van der Kolk, 1988, p. 286).

INSTRUMENTS

There are five basic instruments in psychodrama: the *stage, protagonist, director, auxiliaries/supporting actors,* and *audience.* The *stage* is a space designated for the action—a traditional theater stage, a circle, or simply an area at the end of a room. The function of the stage is to separate the world of drama from the world of real life, an important distinction for participants (Sacks, 1993). Action on the stage is called surplus reality, because it goes beyond what is commonly known. For example, actors can become children or elders, men or women, inanimate objects or feelings. They can play out their dreams and fantasies, go back in time or project themselves into the future. In surplus reality, a Salvadoran refugee can reassemble her family, many members of whom have been lost to her. A Catholic parishioner can talk to the Pope about her disillusionment with the Church and the changes she wants made. A police cadet can swear vociferously at a perpetrator of violence and get to his own fears of being attacked without harming anyone or getting hurt in real life.

The *director* is the producer of the drama. He or she starts with a story or an issue of concern that the group wants to explore. The issue of concern may be represented by a personal story, played by a central actor or *protagonist* who either volunteers or is selected by the group (Buchanan, 1980). The issue of concern can be expressed by a collective story, referred to as a sociodrama, in which the group as a whole explores a community or social issue. In the case of an individual story, the protagonist selects the supporting actors, called *auxiliaries,* because he or she knows the real characters well and has the best sense of who can fulfill the roles. For work with children, Hoey (1997) provides a collection of stuffed animals and puppets that can be used as auxiliaries.

A drama is produced on the spot. It evolves from information provided by the protagonist and from interpretive hunches made by the director and auxiliaries. The director confers with the protagonist about the play's direction and scenes. Throughout, the protagonist has the final say in decisions and is responsible for correcting the director and auxiliaries if the production strays from what is true for him or her.

The *audience* in psychodrama is composed of group members who are active and responsive, unlike spectators of traditional theater. The audience acts as a sounding board for the protagonist and its reverberations can sometimes kindle an emotional release or catharsis. Members of the audience stand ready to assume auxiliary roles as the drama develops such as chorus, extras, a wall, or mentor.

Psychodrama is essentially a group method, sometimes involving large numbers of people. As in any sound group practice, the group leader or director negotiates an agreement with members about the purpose of the group and the responsibilities of those involved, including an understanding about confidentiality. The director promotes a culture of mutual aid and attends simultaneously to the group's development and its productions.

Being theater, psychodrama has great cultural adaptability and can be found in countries across the world. Its methods can be applied to people of all ages and for various purposes: raising consciousness about political and social issues, stabilizing people in situations of trauma and turmoil, revising organizational goals and structures, educating people, and treating interpersonal problems. Psychodrama is not well understood, however, despite its range and history. There are a number of reasons for this: (1) psychodrama is an active, powerful method that makes many therapists trained in talking methods uncomfortable and critical; (2) it has been misused by people without training; (3) it has stood alone, outside of professional schools, universities, and mainstream journals; (4) the media has used its name to refer to strange people and complicated situations such as "psychos" and "drama"; and (5) there is limited empirical evidence substantiating its effectiveness (Blatner, 2000; Fox, 1987).

PHASES OF PSYCHODRAMA

Psychodrama develops in three phases: warm-up, action, and sharing (Z. Moreno, 1969). These phases generally correspond with a curve of emotional expression that peaks in the action phase (Hollander, 2002). However, emotional intensity, along with the time and emphasis of psychodrama sessions, depends on the tolerance of the participants, the setting, and the goals of the group.

For example, clients with considerable emotional hardiness and an aim of psychological insight can generally participate in complex dramas and sessions that last about two hours. The enactment typically starts with scenes from the present, moves to scenes from the past that have the potential to shed light on present day patterns, and returns to present day scenes for application of new learning.

Clients who are emotionally vulnerable, for example those in a crisis or those struggling with mental illness, typically need shorter sessions and a focus on coping. The action portion is generally limited to the present and to practice of specific interpersonal skills. The following is an elaboration of the three phases and their function.

Warm-Up Phase

Professional actors and dancers prepare for roles by stretching, moving, saying lines, and singing scales. Psychodrama actors need similar warm-ups to become spontaneous and prepare for roles. Sometimes group members come to sessions ready to act; sometimes they warm-up naturally as they gather. Other times, they need materials and direction in the form of theater exercises, movement, music, sculpting, drawing, or painting to prepare for action.

It is important to choose and encourage warm-ups that are culturally harmonious, for example, prayer, affirmations, meditation, singing, drumming, teasing, and socializing. If members are unfamiliar with psychodrama, it is appropriate to start with a conversation about the method and then introduce physical activities. Warm-ups are most important in group beginnings, but they are necessary throughout the drama to help players assume new roles and enter new scenes. Warm-ups are used in some groups as a way to start discussion.

Movements, descriptions, metaphors, and feelings expressed in warm-ups are often clues to themes that can be explored further in the action phase (Duffy, 2001).

In a movement warm-up, the director noted that a young woman, usually reticent in the group, was shoving others around, like a bulldozer. Later, when she was chosen to be the protagonist, the director suggested that they start the action with her moving around as the bulldozer again. As she was doing so, he asked if she would describe herself (as the machine) and identify what she was pushing. This was a safe way to begin exploring her situation, leading to further action in the form of scenes with family members (Boria, personal communication, June, 2003).

Action Phase

In the action phase, the story of the protagonist is brought to life on the stage. The example above illustrates how a dilemma and characters can evolve from beginning scenes. In many cases, the protagonist can readily outline for the director what the dilemma is and what he or she wants to achieve. The following is an example of this.

Elizabeth volunteered as a protagonist to test out whether she could manage a task—leaving the alcohol and drug treatment center on a day pass to pick up some clothes from her apartment. To start the drama, the director suggested that Elizabeth set up her apartment. Elizabeth moved some chairs and a table onto the stage, describing the rooms and furnishings as she went along: "This is the kitchen," she said, indicating a portion of the stage. "Here's the countertop." She reached up and hesitated a moment, "Here is the rack where I hang my wine glasses." She walked over to another part of the stage that she designated as the living room. She commented that her roommate had painted the walls a pink color she hated. She brought in chairs for a couch and promptly sat down. "This is where I always drink," she said. And then, "I feel very nervous."

The physical activity of setting up the stage readies the protagonist for the scene. The details of the set help create the protagonist's environment and highlight inherent tensions, influences, and patterns. The example above illustrates how closely feelings and behavior are tied to set and setting, particularly in addictions (Zimberg, 1982). Fortunately Elizabeth experienced her anxieties and her urge to drink within the safety of the stage. She was able to use the stage, further, to test out some alternative actions, such as (1) taking a reliable friend (played by an auxiliary) with her to the apartment and (2) asking a friend to pick up the clothes for her. She recognized that to stay sober, she might need a transitional living situation and later she might have to find a different apartment.

As a drama progresses, scenes of present conflicts can evoke intensely familiar feelings that are linked to conflicts in the past. When these past scenes are enacted the following happens:

> Part of the client's attention is in the past, absorbed in reliving and recounting a distressful experience that has been restimulated by the present context; however, part of the client's attention is also in the present, giving the opportunity to look at it with some distance in perspective and without threat. The protagonist feels the experience as real and true, yet paradoxically and simultaneously is aware that the events are unreal and they can be safely stopped at any moment. (Wiener, 1994, p. 12)

In enactments, the protagonist is encouraged to maximize all expression, using his or her most familiar language to do so. Group members who do not speak the protagonist's language can follow the nonverbal cues until the protagonist is at a point where the dialogue can be interpreted. The protagonist may experience a catharsis—shouting, crying, laughing, dancing—a spontaneous release of deep feelings along with new understanding of the situation. However, in order to produce lasting changes, cognitive and emotional shifts must be integrated and must be accompanied by new behavior and experiences (Dayton, 1994). Final scenes of the action phase can be used for this purpose. Specifically, the protagonist returns to the first scene (where the "trouble" showed up) and enacts it a different way. Sometimes new learning is applied through interaction with group members by setting boundaries or asking for help.

Expressiveness is essential in psychodrama, but so is restraint. Some participants need to learn how to convey their feelings and others need to learn how to modulate them. Psychodrama connects expression to specific interactions and events, so that learning can occur; it does not encourage screaming or hitting a pillow simply for emotional release. Further, acting a certain way on the stage does not mean that the person should or is predisposed to act that way in real life. The protagonist must differentiate which conversations or actions, if any, should be applied. Sometimes the experience of surplus reality on the stage is healing in and of itself.

Sharing and Integration Phase

Zerka Moreno (1969) said, "The only way to repay persons for sharing of themselves is to give of yourself in kind" (p. 238). The final phase of a psychodrama session brings the protagonist back into the folds of the group and allows other members to share how they were touched by the drama. The sharing—in the form of identification with the protagonist, parallel experiences, and personal insights—supports the protagonist in his or her absorption of the experience. Sharing helps group members integrate new discoveries and think about future actions, as well. The director clarifies the purpose of sharing and gently but firmly curtails any tendency toward advice-giving or analysis. It is for the protagonist to determine the significance of the drama and to choose further action.

MAIN TECHNIQUES OF PSYCHODRAMA

The following are the main techniques of psychodrama, used along with the full devices of the theater.

Role Reversal

In role reversal, two people change places embracing how each person views the world through the other's eyes. Playing roles of "you be" and "I'll be" is the essence of empathy. Having empathy is fundamental to developing intimacy in relationships (Klein, 1972). Psychodrama, and role reversal in particular, helps persons develop a broad repertoire of roles, which is associated with social adaptability and psychological health (Blatner, 2000).

A specific function of role reversals in psychodrama is to prepare auxiliaries for their supporting roles. The following illustrates this function.

Characters:	*Daughter*	*Mother*
(1) *in role:*	the protagonist	the auxiliary
(2) *in role reversal:*	auxiliary plays the daughter	the protagonist plays her mother
(3) *return to original places and roles (always)*		

The protagonist and auxiliary physically switch places. The director briefly interviews the protagonist in the mother's role, (e.g., asks her to describe herself in a few words, also to characterize her daughter and the nature of their relationship). The auxiliary observes the presentation of the mother, picking up cues of posture, attitude, and words to use when she resumes that role. When the two reverse back to original roles, they have a brief interchange to let the auxiliary test out her perceptions and to let the protagonist make any needed corrections. Now they are ready to begin the scene.

In addition to using pre-scene role reversals to prepare the cast, directors call for switches during scenes to get authentic dialogue and direction. For example, when the protagonist asks a question that the auxiliary cannot answer, a role reversal allows the protagonist to provide the answer. When the characters change, the auxiliary gives the answer with authority, and the play continues on course.

Role reversals can be done with auxiliaries playing inanimate objects, such as a stuffed animal, a picture on the wall, or a burden on the shoulders. Role reversals can be used to explore universal themes, social situations, and dilemmas such as issues of gender, different generations, culture, power, or scapegoating (Sternberg & Garcia, 2000).

There are some contraindications to the use of role reversal. Karp (1992) cautions:

> Particularly in abusive roles, the protagonist should be protected from playing the role of the perpetrator. The protagonist's job is not to understand why the abuse happened, but to concentrate on venting the feelings that have occurred because of the abuse. (p. 109)

The following vignette illustrates a problematic role reversal that took place at an alcohol treatment center for adults. The example is included to demonstrate the power of psychodrama and the necessity of solid training for directors.

In a warm-up involving newspapers, Natalie made a paper sailboat that she pushed back and forth in front of her. Noting this, the director asked whether the boat had some meaning that she wanted to explore in action. Natalie was hesitant. She was not sure she wanted to go aboard the boat because the sea was rough. The director encouraged her and checked with the group to assure its support. Natalie gave a few details about the boat and then stepped aboard. Asked who was on the boat, she said, "My father." She reluctantly picked someone from the group to play her father and then reluctantly role reversed. To help her warm up to the role, the director asked her to move around as the father, to describe himself—what was he wearing? She froze, dropped out of role and said, "He isn't wearing anything."

The implications of sexual abuse were clear. In retrospect, the director was inattentive to the protagonist's ambivalence about doing the scene. She might have explored the "rough seas," for example, or asked Natalie directly about her hesitancy. Even so, psychodrama sessions are unpredictable and directors need to be able to think on their feet. Using her knowledge of theatrical and therapeutic strategies, the director in this particular drama pictures the following alternatives:

1. Asking Natalie if there is a safe place for her to go and, if so, directing her to that haven until the boat returns to shore. Following that, helping Natalie rehearse some steps she can take next.
2. Suggesting that perhaps there are people in Natalie's life who can "rescue" her from the boat. Directing an enactment of the rescue. Natalie picks auxiliaries to play specific rescuers.
3. Using artistic license and her authority as director to manage the scene. Saying to the father, for example, "Sir, go put on your clothes. You have no right to behave this way. This is your daughter."
4. Acknowledging the trauma and suggesting a scene where Natalie can practice new ways of dealing with her memories other than cutting herself and drinking.
5. Moving to the sharing portion of the session, if the protagonist does not wish to continue the action. Guiding members to share their reactions to the disclosure rather than asking further questions or making new disclosures themselves.

The Double

The double is an auxiliary who plays the part of the protagonist—the part not readily available to consciousness. Initially, the double assumes the physical poses and movements of the protagonist from a position slightly back from the protagonist's side. The physical state often gives clues to the emotional state. The double can be supportive by physical presence or encouraging words, can make observations, raise feeling, or provoke or amplify specific feelings. The double uses the first person in speech, but other actors do not respond unless the protagonist picks up the words and says them. Doubling is a complex assignment, requiring great sensitivity and judgment. The double must behave in accord with the protagonist to gain acceptance, but must stir the protagonist to consider new viewpoints, expression, and action (Leveton, 2001).

Mirroring

An auxiliary steps into the protagonist's place, allowing the protagonist to view himself or herself in the scene from the outside. This technique is especially useful when protagonists get stuck in repetitive patterns. Mirroring provides them a different perspective and distance from the emotional intensity of the scene. As a result, they can often return to action with greater energy and clarity.

Soliloquy

This is a theatrical aside, spoken as if the protagonist were alone. A soliloquy reveals inner thoughts and feelings that have not been expressed directly to other actors or the audience.

Concretizing

This technique gives substance to abstract ideas and feelings; it makes them concrete. Vague or obscure issues are difficult to work with unless they are translated into objects with specific details or into scenes with specific people. If protagonists need to be indirect because of safety issues or cultural norms, metaphors can provide concrete images from which to work.

Personification

This is a type of concretization that brings feelings, images, and objects to life. For example, "a knot in my stomach," "a sea of shame," or "a monkey on my back" can be enacted by auxiliaries. Pets, pictures on the wall, and other objects can be given voice with which to explore and amplify a scene.

The Empty Chair

A chair is set out as a focus point. Members of the group visualize persons or objects on the chair, usually representative of some concern or unfinished business. The chair can be used alone, that is, group members can direct statements to the imagined person there or the chair can be occupied by auxiliaries with whom further work can be accomplished.

Future Projection

The protagonist enacts a future situation as if she or he were there. This technique offers new visions and provides a way to check out choices or practice skills that are required.

Dream Projection

Starting with preparation for sleep, the protagonist enacts a dream, complete with scene-setting and interaction with essential auxiliaries. Subsequently, the protagonist reenacts the dream, changing it as she or he wishes it to be. Repair and retraining occurs through enacting this preferred dream. Meaning is left to the protagonist. No analysis or interpretation is suggested, although other group members may share similar stories or points of identification with the dreamer.

Some of the techniques, such as the empty chair, role reversal, and future projection, can be used in individual therapy (Vander May, 1981; Fowler, 1992). Some therapists like to bring in trained auxiliaries to assist in sessions. This is not necessary, however, as clients can move back and forth to play both themselves and other roles. It is advisable for the counselor or therapist to remain as the director, rather than to take on auxiliary roles.

EXAMPLES OF PSYCHODRAMA IN DIFFERENT SETTINGS

The following are descriptions or case studies that illustrate how psychodrama may be adapted to groups in different settings.

Alcohol and Drug Treatment Group

This psychodrama session took place in a residential center, with 18 group members present. The director led the group in a movement warm-up and then put out a variety of art materials. She asked the participants to draw themselves and the drugs that had become troublesome in their lives. Some people immediately started selecting materials. One man said that it was like kindergarten; a few said that they could not draw. The director encouraged them all to try sketching—simple line drawings would be fine. When they finished, the director asked them to show their drawings and say a few words about them. As individuals held up their sketches, other members responded appreciatively; they identified with the situations and the feelings portrayed. One man, called Ephraim, drew himself isolated in a dark room with a bottle on the table in front of him; Joelle drew herself under a spectrum of colors, beginning with bright ones and ending with black. Peter, an adolescent, drew himself "wired," with hair sticking straight up, big bloodshot eyes, and a wide smile. He was smoking a huge joint and snorting coke; he had a beer in one hand and a shot of whisky ready on the bar. His drawing drew a big reaction and group members started advising him about drugs he could use to prevent his being strung out. The director stopped them after a minute, observing that they seemed to be playing pharmacist—prescribing drugs to counteract drug effects. What did this mean for them now, in terms of their goals? After some discussion, the director asked group members to draw second pictures—of themselves in recovery, not using drugs.

In contrast to his isolation in the first picture, Ephraim drew himself outside, jogging along the river with a friend. Peter, however, drew himself in a priest's cassock holding the BIG BOOK of AA. The word, BORING was written at the top, along with "Keep it simple, stupid." Again, Peter's drawing brought a strong reaction. He expressed the skepticism that many group members felt about life without drugs—dull and monastic, without zest. Members started to mourn the loss of life without drugs. Others talked about the gains of sobriety, many of which were depicted in their drawings.

The director asked for volunteers to bring their pictures to action. Ephraim volunteered and began to set the stage for the first scene (essentially a kitchen table, chair, and a bottle). With the director standing by, he established the time of day, sounds, other details of the room, and how long he had lived at the apartment. The director moved off stage and darkened the room. Ephraim then sat down in front of a very quiet audience. After a long pause, the director suggested a soliloquy, and the protagonist spoke about the misery, loneliness, and hopelessness he felt. He was at a critical point where he would either commit suicide or get help. The director moved in and suggested that Ephraim enact the telephone call that brought him into treatment. Together they advanced the time (done typically by walking around and counting off time periods) and moved to the next drawing/scene, which took place in the park along the river. Ephraim chose a group member as his friend and jogging mate. The director suggested that they run several times around the circular resident hall outside of the meeting room. The runners took off, then burst back into the group room, out of breath and full of energy. The group applauded spontaneously.

Following the drama, the group members settled into a sharing of enjoyable and healthy experiences—such as seeing the morning light, feeling more energy, eating nutritious meals, beginning to see their family again—since getting off alcohol and drugs. They did not deny the difficulty or the dedication it would take to maintain these new patterns, but expressed a sense of hope and renewal.

A Third Grade Class

A teacher and a psychodrama director collaborated on two projects, a social studies unit on the Vikings and a reading project, which is described in the following text.

The director instructed the children to think of their favorite character from a book they had read. Then they were to get quietly into that character's book, on the bookshelf. The children helped construct a bookshelf out of a double row of little stools—then they squeezed in together. The director continued that at night when it was dark the characters came out one by one to play. She darkened the room and one child immediately jumped out as Pippy Longstocking. Other characters followed—Merlin, Ramona Quimby, the dog Sounder, and so on. As more characters appeared and the action got a little chaotic, the teacher spontaneously pulled out her flute and played softly (a norm she had established in her class to bring quiet); she and the director suggested that the characters on the stage could play together until they heard the music. Then, they would freeze so that a new character could come out and have center stage for a few minutes. The children had a wonderful time, imaginatively as the characters and interpersonally as a class.

Training for Mental Health Clinicians and Counselors

A student in a clinical practice class raised questions about an intake session that involved a pregnant teen, her boyfriend, and the boyfriend's mother. The student was uncomfortable with the standard list of intake questions and did not know how to respond to three people at the same time. She was inclined to direct her attention to the couple. Using psychodrama methods, the teacher asked the student to set up the interviewing room and to choose three classmates to play the family members. The student then modeled each character's physical position and gave three descriptive words for each. As the auxiliaries took their places, a picture of family relationships emerged: the couple sat close together, the young man being protective of his "very pale" girlfriend; the mother sat off to the side, "wanting to give her opinion, but trying not to intrude." Action, in the form of a short vignette, provided further information: although the young man left school and was not working (identified as the problem by the mother), he had cared for his partner during several hospitalizations. And, it turned out that both sets of parents were supportive—they alternated weekends for having the couple at their homes.

Use of psychodrama in this class helped students make a systemic assessment that focused on family strengths. As a consequence, students were able to identify possible approaches that would help the extended family reduce tension around health care and financial responsibilities.

Social Action and Community Development

Brazilian director Boal (1985) is best known for using theater to accomplish political and social action. Enlisting people from the community to perform scenes from their daily lives, Boal raises consciousness about social conditions and provokes change. Similar social action and community development projects are taking place in many countries of the world.

Bangladesh is the most densely populated country in the world. In 2004, several psychodrama directors from the United States collaborated with the United Theatre for Social Action in Bangladesh to conduct a National Therapeutic Theater Workshop. Participating in the workshop were social activists—mostly young people employed in nongovernmental organizations (NGOs)—who were already working with school children to produce plays based on their life experiences. The workshop brought together psychodramatists, NGO staff, directors, playwrights, drama critics, and university professors; it laid the groundwork for a psychodrama institute in Bangladesh and promoted interest in the educational, therapeutic, and social use of theater (Herb Propper, personal communication, 2004).

EFFICACY OF PSYCHODRAMA

Moreno devised a range of empirical and action tests to measure social interaction, to compare methods, and to test spontaneity, creativity, and role capacity. Calling psychodrama "the science that explores the truth by means of action methods" (Moreno & Moreno, 1975, p. 191), he recommended behavioral rather than personality tests to determine outcomes. His advice was not always heeded, however, and validation of psychodrama's effectiveness has been hampered over the years by a number of factors: (1) the majority of studies are descriptive; (2) the definition of psychodrama is inconsistent among and between studies, varying from "classical" to role play and a range of other experiential and expressive methods; (3) many studies do not outline the credentials of the directors or the specific methods employed; (4) psychodrama and its techniques are often used in conjunction with other therapeutic approaches to treat multiple symptoms, making it difficult to isolate particular influences; and (5) studies are limited in sample size and lack follow-up data (D'Amato & Dean, 1988; Kipper, 1978).

Outcome Studies

Behavioral outcome measures of psychodrama are increasingly available. Kellerman (1987), who reviewed 23 outcome studies from 1952 to 1985 that fit the criteria for experimental design and for classical psychodrama, concluded that psychodrama constitutes a valid alternative to other therapeutic approaches. For example, subjects in a residential facility for the treatment of alcohol abuse reported increased activity, trust, and emotional stability after four, three-hour weekly psychodrama sessions (Wood, Del Nuovo, Bucky, Schein, & Michalik, 1979). In correctional institutions, psychodrama groups have been shown to improve basic educational skills (Melnick, 1984), adjustment to prison life (Stallone, 1993), and sense of interpersonal adequacy (Schramski, Feldman, Harvey, & Holiman, 1984). In a community project for mothers identified as abusive to their children, use of psychodrama positively affected their attitudes of self-acceptance, self-control, responsibility, and socialization (White, Rosenblatt, Love, & Little, 1982). In a short-term residential center that based its treatment on psychodrama theory and techniques, clients with post-traumatic stress disorder (PTSD), and with anxiety and mood disorders reported enhanced well-being and a significant reduction of symptoms (Klontz, Wolf, & Bivens, 2001). An Indian study of male patients with primary depression revealed that psychodrama group therapy after 24 weeks was a reliable and effective means of reducing participants' levels of depression, being significantly more effective than conventional psychiatric treatment of the same period (Rezaeian, Sen, & Mazumdar, 1997).

A study evaluating the effectiveness of psychodrama groups with middle-school girls, who had experienced at least seven traumatic events, suggested a significant decrease in the participants' self-reported difficulties of anxiety/depression and withdrawn behavior, as compared to the control group. Interviews with the girls highlighted the value of the group, particularly the mutual support, development of coping techniques, and increased sense of self-efficacy (Carbonell & Parteleno-Barehmi, 1999).

Promising Studies

A few qualitative studies are available, notably a rigorous analysis of psychodrama sessions conducted by Italian director Boria (2001) for the purpose of elaborating psychodrama process. There is a great potential in qualitative studies, including analysis of Moreno's verbatim records (located in Special Collections at Harvard University Medical Library).

Studies from other fields, such as neuroscience and psychobiology, may be the best sources of evidence for the efficacy of psychodrama. Studies in the field of trauma and depression, cited earlier, demonstrate the value of spontaneity and action in retraining. Studies by Rossi (2002) provide evidence that enriching life experiences, novelty, and physical activity can activate new brain growth, including a reframing of memories. Cross-discipline studies of psychodrama are highly recommended; these should be conducted in education, community, and treatment arenas.

REFERENCES

Blatner, A. (2000). *Foundations of psychodrama: History, theory and practice* (4th ed.). New York: Springer.

Boal, A. (1985). *Theatre of the oppressed.* New York: Theatre Communications Groups.

Boria, G. (2001). *Il percorso psicodrammatico di Anna e di Maria.* Milan, Italy: Studio di Psicodrama.

Buchanan, D. (1980). The central concern model: A framework for structuring psychodramatic production. *Journal of Group Psychotherapy, Psychodrama and Sociometry, 33,* 47-62.

Carbonell, D.M. & Parteleno-Barehmi, C. (1999). Psychodrama groups for girls coping with trauma. *International Journal of Group Psychotherapy, 49*(3), 285-306.

D'Amato, R.K. & Dean, R.S. (1988). Psychodrama research—Therapy and theory: A critical analysis of an arrested modality. *Psychology in the Schools, 25,* 305-314.

Dayton, T. (1994). *The drama within: Psychodrama and experiential therapy.* Deerfield Beach, FL: Health Communications.

Duffy, T.K. (2001). White gloves and cracked vases: How metaphors help group workers construct new perspectives and responses. *Social Work with Groups, 24*(3/4), 89-99.

Fowler, R. (1992). *Using psychodrama in individual counseling and psychotherapy.* Psychodrama thesis. Australian and New Zealand Psychodrama Association. Wellington: Fowler.

Fox, J. (1987). *The essential Moreno: Writings on psychodrama, group method and spontaneity by J.L. Moreno.* New York: Springer Publishers.

Hoey, B. (1997). *Who calls the tune: A psychodramatic approach to child therapy.* New York: Routledge.

Hollander, C. (2002). A process for psychodrama training: The Hollander psychodrama curve. *International Journal of Action Methods, 54*(4), 147-157. (Original work published 1978.)

Holmes, P., Karp, M., & Watson, M. (Eds.). (1994). *Psychodrama since Moreno: Innovations in theory and practice.* New York: Routledge.

Karp, M. (1992). Psychodrama and Picallili. In P. Holmes & M. Karp (Eds.), *Psychodrama, inspiration and technique*. New York: Routledge.

Kellerman, P.F. (1987). Outcome research in classical psychodrama. *Small Group Behavior, 18*(4), 459-469.

Kipper, D.A. (1978). Trends in research on the effectiveness of psychodrama: Retrospect and prospect. *Journal of Group Psychotherapy, Psychodrama & Sociometry, 31*, 5-18.

Klontz, B.T., Wolf, E.M., & Bivens, A. (2001). Psychodrama, skill training, and role playing. *International Journal of Action Methods, 53*(3/4), 119-135.

Leveton, E. (2001). *A clinician's guide to psychodrama* (3rd ed.). New York: Springer.

Marineau, R.F. (1989). *Jacob Levy Moreno 1889-1974*. London: Routledge.

Melnick, M. (1984). Skills through drama: The use of professional theater techniques in the treatment and education of prison and ex-offender populations. *Journal of Group Psychotherapy, Psychodrama and Sociometry, 37*, 104-116.

Moreno, J.L. (1943, January 14). *Notes on lecture at City College: Difference between psychodrama and psychoanalysis*. Unpublished Manuscript. Boston, MA: Harvard University Medical School.

Moreno, J.L. (1953). *Who shall survive? Foundations of sociometry, group psychotherapy and sociodrama*. Beacon, NY: Beacon House. (Original work published 1934 with the subtitle A new approach to the problems of human relations.)

Moreno, J.L. (1957). *The first book on group psychotherapy* (3rd ed.). Beacon, NY: Beacon House. (Original work published 1932; Part I published 1931.)

Moreno, J.L. (1968). Universal peace in our time. *Group Psychotherapy, 21*, 175-179.

Moreno, J.L. (1983). *Theatre of spontaneity*. Ambler, PA: Beacon House. (Original work published 1947.)

Moreno, J.L. (1985). *Psychodrama* (7th ed., Vol. 1). Ambler, PA: Beacon, NY: Beacon House. (Original work published 1946.)

Moreno, J.L. & Moreno, Z.T. (1975). *Psychodrama: Foundations of psychotherapy* (2nd ed., Vol. 2). Beacon, NY: Beacon House. (Original work published 1959.)

Moreno, Z.T. (1969). Psychodramatic rules, techniques and adjunctive methods. In J.L. Moreno & Z.T. Moreno, *Psychodrama, Vol. 3*. (pp. 233-246). Beacon, NY: Beacon House. (Original work published 1965.)

Rezaeian, M.P., Sen, A.K., & Mazumdar, D.P. (1997). The usefulness of psychodrama in the treatment of depressed patients. *Indian Journal of Clinical Psychology, 24*(1), 82-88.

Rossi, E.L. (2002). *The psychobiology of gene expression*. New York: Norton & Co.

Sacks, J. (1993). Psychodrama. In H. Kaplan & B. Sadock (Eds.), *Comprehensive group psychotherapy* (3rd ed., pp. 214-228). Baltimore: Williams &Wilkins.

Schramski, T.G., Feldman, C.A., Harvey, D.R., & Holiman, M.A. (1984). A comparative evaluation of group treatment in an adult correctional facility. *Journal of Group Psychotherapy, Psychodrama, & Sociometry, 36*, 133-147.

Stallone, T.M. (1993). The effects of psychodrama on inmates within a structured residential behavior modification program. *Journal of Group Psychotherapy, Psychodrama, & Sociometry, 46*(1), 24-31.

Sternberg, P. & Garcia, A. (2000). *Sociodrama: Who's in your shoes?* (2nd ed.). Westport, CT: Praeger.

van der Kolk, B.A. (1988). The biologic response to psychic trauma. In F.M. Ochberg (Ed.), *Post-traumatic therapy and victims of violence* (pp. 25-38). New York: Brunner/Mazel.

van der Kolk, B., & van der Hart, O. (1995). The intrusive past: The flexibility of memory and the engraving of trauma. In C. Caruth (Ed.), *Explorations in memory* (pp. 158-182). Baltimore, MD: John Hopkins University Press.

Vander May, J. (1981). *Psychodrama a deux: Practical applications of psychodrama to individual counseling.* Grand Rapids, MI: Pine Rest Christian Hospital.

White, E.W., Rosenblatt, E., Love, A., & Little, D. (1982). *Psychodrama and life skills: A treatment alternative in child abuse.* Unpublished manuscript, Toronto Center for Psychodrama and Sociometry.

Wiener, D. (1994). *Rehearsals for growth: Theater improvisation for psychotherapists.* New York: Norton.

Wood, D., Del Nuovo, A., Bucky, S.F., Schein, S., & Michalik, M. (1979). Psychodrama with an alcohol abuser population. *Group Psychotherapy, Psychodrama, & Sociometry, 32,* 75-88.

Zimberg, S. (1982). *The clinical management of alcoholism.* New York: Brunner/Mazel.

Chapter 7

Dance/Movement Therapy

Irma Dosamantes-Beaudry

THE CREATIVE ARTS THERAPIES' FIELD AND DANCE/MOVEMENT THERAPY

The creative arts therapies' field encompasses arts-based therapies (art therapy, dance therapy, drama therapy, music therapy, and poetry therapy) that initially emerged in this country during the 1960s. Although each of these creative art therapies gradually acquired its own unique professional identity because of the unique art medium that it used, all shared certain assumptions about the use of arts media as therapy: (1) that arts' media could be used by trained creative arts therapists as therapeutic modalities and (2) that the creative therapeutic process that was set into motion by creative arts therapies could promote self-generativity, self-integration, and communal transformation (Landy, 1997; Dosamantes-Beaudry, 2003).

Rediscovering the Ancient Healing Role of Dance

The emergence of dance/movement therapy (DMT) as a unique therapeutic modality and practice in this country during the 1960s, represents a modern day re-discovery of the healing role of dance recognized for thousands of years by tribal communities that have continued to incorporate dance in their sacred rituals. Some of the healing functions served by dance in these communities include (1) helping members mediate unknown and uncontrollable forces

Introduction to Alternative and Complementary Therapies
© 2008 by The Haworth Press, Taylor & Francis Group. All rights reserved.
doi:10.1300/5987_07   *153*

within themselves and their environment, (2) offering a safe way to act out negative or deviant emotions and behaviors, (3) providing a means of enacting changes in adopted role or status, (4) helping individuals release emotions arising from experienced conflict or pent-up frustration, and (5) reaffirming each member's inclusiveness in his or her cultural group. In sum, within tribal communities, dance has served to restore individual and communal emotional balance and to reinforce the social order of the community (Hanna, 1979).

DMT not only represents an embodied, unfolding, creative, psychodynamic therapeutic process but because it is a practice that is conducted primarily by female therapists, this body-based psychotherapeutic modality directly challenges our Western society's patriarchal Cartesian view of the body (Aalten, 1997; Davis, 1997). Once the carnal genie was let out of the bottle, the energy and instinctive wisdom of the body was able to rejoin human consciousness (Dosamantes-Beaudry, 1999). By acknowledging that body and spirit are inexorably intertwined, a reconciliation of previously seemingly incompatible polarities (e.g., body and mind, male and female, sacred and profane) became possible (Dosamantes-Beaudry, 2001). At present the vast majority of American DMT practitioners continue to be female.

AMERICAN DANCE THERAPY ASSOCIATION

During the 1960s under the leadership of Marian Chace, second generation dance therapists set out to organize a national professional organization, the American Dance Therapy Association (ADTA), to represent the interests of its members and clients. This professional organization set goals and objectives for itself that were similar in scope to those set by larger clinical professional organizations. Since its inception, the ADTA has helped to (1) set educational, professional, and ethical standards of practice, (2) underwrite an annual national conference, (3) publish a professional journal, titled *American Journal of Dance Therapy,* and produce a national newsletter.

The educational effectiveness of this organization can be gauged by the number of academic institutions that currently offer graduate DMT training in the United States and abroad and the extent to which DMT has been exported and is practiced internationally. Some of the countries in which DMT is currently practiced include Argentina,

Australia, Belgium, Brazil, Canada, China, Denmark, Egypt, England, Finland, France, Italy, Germany, Japan, Korea, Mexico, Norway, Russia, Scotland, Spain, Sweden, Switzerland, and Taiwan (Pallaro, 1995). How DMT is defined and practiced in each of these nations will need to be determined by cross-cultural empirical studies conducted by dance therapists in the future.

DEFINITION, PREMISES, AND PRACTITIONERS OF DMT

In 1974, the American Dance Therapy Association defined DMT as the psychotherapeutic use of movement as a process that furthered the emotional and physical integration of the individual (Bunney, 1980). The premises upon which the practice of DMT is founded include the following:

1. Emotional well-being is reflected in the integration of body and mind. Emotional disorder is manifested in the dissociation of body from mind.
2. Body-movement is a medium through which an individual can experience, express, and communicate elements of experience that are not readily communicable through verbal means and tend to be less conscious.
3. When individuals move spontaneously, their movement reveals something about their emotional state of the moment as well as the manner in which they ward off the expression of particular affects.
4. When individuals move in relation to one or more persons, their movement reflects something about the emotional nature of their ongoing relationship and the way they defend or protect themselves against others emotionally.
5. It is possible for an individual to explore intrapsychic and interpersonal emotional concerns or problems in the safe, potential play space that is created over time within the context of the therapeutic collaborative relationship that is established with a trained dance therapist. (Dosamantes-Alperson, 1981, pp. 4-5)

DMT was pioneered by several modern dancers: Marian Chace, Liljan Espenak, and Franziska Boas on the East Coast and Mary Whitehouse, Trudi Schoop, and Alma Hawkins on the West Coast (Bartenieff, 1972). As practitioners trained in Western modern dance, these DMT pioneers shared a belief in the healing potential of individual spontaneous expressive body movement and body self-awareness.

Because many second generation dance therapists in the United States have also been trained as psychotherapists, their interdisciplinary background as dancers and psychotherapists has helped to forge an interdisciplinary, hybrid identity for DMT. So at present, DMT as a professional practice synthesizes the bodily awareness, individual expressiveness, spontaneity, and creativity of Western modern dance with some of the clinical methods and theoretical concepts of various schools of contemporary Western psychotherapy. Today a wide variety of psychodynamic DMT approaches such as "Chace," "Jungian," or "Psychoanalytic" and others are practiced (Dosamantes-Beaudry, 1997). Despite the theoretical differences that underlie these approaches, most dance therapists share the concept of the use of body movement as a means of facilitating a creative, psychotherapeutic process that culminates in body-mind integration as well as self and group transformation. What distinguishes the practice of DMT from most verbal forms of psychotherapy is its direct and extensive use of body movement as a medium for emotional self-expression and a means of communication with others.

Some goals shared in common by dance therapists include (1) increased body-self awareness, (2) expansion of one's expressive movement range, (3) increased spontaneity and openness to experience, (4) increased awareness of personal and interpersonal areas of conflict, (5) increased capacity to draw associations and meaning from one's movement experience, (6) increased application of insights derived from the DMT context to the client's lived experience and to relationships outside of the therapeutic arena.

DMT AS A CREATIVE, PSYCHODYNAMIC THERAPEUTIC PROCESS

What distinguishes DMT from mechanistic "body therapies" is the greater attention paid by dance therapists to the unfolding creative, psychodynamic therapeutic process and the derivation of the symbolic meaning contained in the movement metaphors that DMT clients generate spontaneously over the course of the therapeutic process. The dance therapist does not offer a set of exercises simply to effect certain mechanical changes in the physical structure, posture, and actions of the client. Also, he/she always takes into consideration the emotional impact that any physical intervention is likely to have upon a particular client who possesses a unique emotional and cultural history. Also, the client is mindful of the fact that the therapeutic DMT process that evolves over time takes place within an intersubjective space that continually shifts and is transformed and revised over time by both the client and the dance therapist.

EMPLOYMENT SETTINGS

Today one finds dance therapists employed at a variety of clinical settings that include hospitals, outpatient mental health clinics, correctional facilities, day-care centers, homeless shelters, shelters for battered women, alternative medicine clinics, holistic healing centers, pain clinics, wellness centers, counseling centers, and schools. Some teach at universities and colleges and conduct research. Many experienced dance therapists also conduct private practices (Duggan, Bell, Orleans, Wexler, Bennett, & Greenberg, 1979). Client populations served by dance therapists include clients who differ in age, experience, and varying degrees of emotional coherence, and capacity for self-regulation. Some are mentally challenged or physically disabled; others are terminally ill or suffer from various kinds of psychosomatic and immunological disorders. Dance therapists also work with victims of domestic abuse, with homeless people, and with individuals who are enrolled in illness prevention programs (Dosamantes-Beaudry, 1999).

VARIETY OF DMT TREATMENT APPROACHES

The DMT approaches developed by American dance therapists have been largely influenced by the zeitgeist of their time (Levy, 1988). Thus, during DMT's pioneering era which extended from the 1940s to the 1960s, the influence of Western modern dance was most keenly felt. Each pioneer developed his or her own unique brand of

DMT based upon his or her own personality, dance training, his or her unique understanding of the role of dance in maintaining a person's well being, and the emotional functional level of the clients with whom he or she worked.

Later, during the 1970s and through the 1980s, dance therapists were strongly influenced by the Humanistic Psychology Movement of the time which in turn gave rise to "gestalt" and "experiential" DMT approaches. Since the 1980s, psychodynamic approaches founded upon psychoanalytic and analytic theories that placed greater emphasis upon the unfolding psychodynamics, unconscious processes, and the intersubjective field in which the client-therapist relationship was transacted gained popularity (Dosamantes-Beaudry, 1999).

With adult clients, the psychodynamic DMT process generally appears to move through the following distinctive phases:

Phase One: Introduction and Assessment of Appropriateness of DMT As a Therapeutic Modality

During the first DMT session, clients describe the existential predicament that has led them to seek DMT treatment. The dance therapist listens and observes how they present their concerns (verbally and nonverbally). At some point, the dance therapist encourages them to explore some aspect of their immediate subjective experience through a movement process that is facilitated by the dance therapist. Toward the end of the session, clients are given the opportunity to verbally share some aspect of their moved experience with the dance therapist.

The term *potential play space* refers to a psychologically safe therapeutic environment where clients feel free to engage in pretend play and to give outward expression to their inner symbolic life through spontaneously generated movement metaphors, images, and words. During the initial phases of DMT, the dance therapist begins to facilitate the emergence of a potential play space by listening carefully to the client's presenting concerns, by attending to how the client communicates in verbal and nonverbal ways, and by gauging and providing the degree of movement structure he or she estimates a particular client might need to move freely in a self-directed, spontaneous, and explorative manner. The client's movement experience becomes the focus of what is discussed between them. Within the context of DMT groups, clients also have the opportunity to engage in interactive movement with other group members.

Early DMT sessions also serve a useful assessment function. Both verbal and nonverbal movement components of a session allow the dance therapist to: (1) assess the functional emotional developmental level of a given client, (2) gauge the client's tolerance for regression without becoming emotionally overwhelmed and fragmented while moving, (3) outline whether or not the client is likely to benefit from DMT and if the answer to (3) is yes, (4) determine whether the particular client would benefit most from being seen individually or within the context of a group. Such an initial assessment is critical in order to determine the best therapeutic course of action to be followed with a particular client.

The potential play space that a dance therapist facilitates from the outset of treatment in order to encourage spontaneity in thought and action also seems to induce a state of regression in clients. The term *regression* refers to a person's capacity to temporarily return to earlier modes of perceiving, thinking, and being (Dosamantes-Beaudry, 1998, 2003). Regressive states can be characterized as either adaptive or maladaptive. When clients undergo an *adaptive, benign,* or *voluntary* form of regression they are able to maintain some degree of emotional distance from their subjective experience and the capacity to be self-reflective. By contrast, when clients undergo an *involuntary, maladaptive,* or *structural* regression they experience such regression as an intrusive and unwanted event because it seems to come upon them suddenly and unexpectedly and they experience themselves as having no control over it. Clients who undergo a structural regression tend to fuse consensual and subjective realities and the structural intactness of their sense of self (i.e., their mode of thinking, their sense of time, space, and body-self) becomes dramatically altered and impaired. A structural regression can therefore be a very confusing and frightening experience for a client.

Clinical Example

The following clinical example illustrates how an initial session was used by a dance therapist to assess a client's emotional developmental level, his capacity for benign regression, and to provide a recommendation for appropriate treatment.

John was referred to me for a private practice consultation by a psychiatrist who was interested in determining whether he might benefit from DMT and whether he could be seen individually on an outpatient basis. The referring psychiatrist mentioned that John loved to dance. He wondered whether the medium of movement might be the best way to initiate a therapeutic dialogue with him.

John showed up at my office-studio dressed skimpily and barefooted though it was winter and rather chilly outside, indicating a degree of obliviousness to his physical well-being. He let me know that he had recently undergone an "emotional breakdown," which he blamed entirely upon his father. He characterized his father as an emotionally distant, critical, and demanding man. He also mentioned that he loved to dance. When I asked him whether he would like to move, he eagerly responded in the affirmative. As he began to move in a self-directed way in the movement studio, I noticed that he repeatedly lunged across the studio space in seeming wild abandon. He repeatedly flung his body against the hard walls of the movement studio without any apparent concern for any injuries he might inflict upon himself. Based upon his expressive movement behavior, I determined that at this time John was out of touch with his own bodily felt experience and lacked a clear sense of his own body boundaries. Experientially he merged with whatever environment he came into contact. In sum, his behavior was characteristic of someone who had recently undergone a psychotic break.

I surmised that some time prior to his coming to see me he had undergone an involuntarily regression and returned to an earlier state of being, perceiving, and thinking. Because of his lack of self-awareness and because for him ordinary consensual reality and subjective experience had become fused, it was not possible for him at this time to adapt the emotional distance that would have allowed him to make sense of the process that he was undergoing. John had become emotionally overwhelmed by his involuntary regressive experience. His judgment and capacity for emotional self-regulation in the outside world had become impaired.

In my opinion as long as John remained enmeshed in the throes of a structural regression, he could inadvertently physically injure himself. Therefore, I informed the referring psychiatrist that I believed John could benefit from individual psychodynamic DMT because he readily expressed himself through spontaneous movement and because DMT could offer him a means to regain an embodied sense of self and to acquire a clearer sense of his own body boundaries. However, because John was in the throes of an involuntary regression, such a therapeutic process would need to be conducted only within the context of an emotionally supportive closed environment with a dance therapist who understood the psychodynamics involved in the regression-reintegration process (Dosamantes-Beaudry, 1998). A physically closed environment that offered John the opportunity to establish a potential play space with an experienced dance therapist would afford John an opportunity to restore a sense of his body self, body boundaries, cohesive sense of self, and emotional equilibrium.

Phase Two: Developing Trust and Discovering Receptive and Active Kinds of Movement

Once it has been determined that a particular client can benefit from DMT, the creation of a potential play space becomes the primary task of this phase of the treatment process. The dance therapist accomplishes this by showing him or her self to be reliable, consistent, and expert in what he or she does over the duration of the treatment process. During the second phase of the treatment process, it becomes the therapist's responsibility to act as an effective container for the client's emotional reactions to the process, to provide the proper level of movement structure he or she estimates the client needs to function comfortably within the treatment setting, and to introduce the client to two kinds of movement experiences that dance therapists use in their work.

I have previously referred to these two kinds of movement as "active" and "receptive" (Dosamantes-Alperson, 1979). Receptive movement is a movement that takes place while the movers are in a receptive state of consciousness and their attention is relaxed and maintained upon their own internal sensations, emotions, and images. In contrast, active movement takes place while movers are in an active state of consciousness and their attention is focused outwardly upon the kinds of movement interactions that they forge with other people and with other external objects or events.

Within an individual DMT context, when clients whose eyes are open begin to move freely and spontaneously, they start to perceive the emotional movement patterns they tend to favor which characterize their own unique movement style. If they move within the context of a DMT group, clients also acquire some sense of how they interact with others nonverbally. They begin to notice the kinds of emotional movement patterns they resort to and rely upon when moving with different members of the group.

In either individual or group DMT, clients also have an opportunity to explore their internal self-experience in a nonverbal way. They do so by shifting from an active to a receptive state of consciousness. This is accomplished by closing their eyes, becoming quiet, and attending inwardly to their ongoing sensory experience and spontaneously emergent images. The sensations and images that surface to their awareness generally bring to the forefront some significant psychodynamic theme they happen to be working on. By accessing their self-experience through nonverbal modalities, clients begin to acquire the capacity to bridge less conscious with more conscious aspects of their self-experience.

Phase Three: Embodying Polarized Aspects of Internal Symbolic Experience

As trust in the DMT situation and in the dance therapist deepens, it becomes possible for clients to risk drawing deeper connections between their moved experience and the symbols that emerge from their own imagination. The psychodynamic themes that surface reflect deeper kinds of emotional conflicts that the clients are struggling with in their lives.

When clients have developed a sense of trust in the treatment process and have become acquainted with the use of "receptive" and "active" kinds of movement, they are able to begin exploring more difficult, polarized aspects of their internal symbolic experience. Sessions that occur during this phase seem to follow a predictable pattern: (1) clients describe (verbally or nonverbally) some residual reactions they had to a previous session, (2) the dance therapist tunes into the predominant psychodynamic theme being expressed by them, (3) the dance therapist focuses clients' attention upon various polarized aspects of their subjective experience, (4) clients determine those aspects of their subjective experience they will embody and explore further through self-directed, spontaneous movement, and (5) clients verbally share aspects of their moved experience with the dance therapist.

Clinical Example

The following clinical example illustrates how a professional dancer worked to synthesize polarized aspects of her self-experience.

As a professional dancer, Joanna performed technically difficult movements brilliantly on stage, but in an emotionally detached way that gave her performance a robotic, detached appearance. When she attempted to move spontaneously without any preconceived notion of how she should move within the DMT context, she initially found herself extremely frightened and unable to move altogether.

Over time Joanna began to recover and to reclaim the emotional excitement that originally drew her to the field of dance before parental pressure drove her to become a professional dancer so that she could financially support her entire family. Joanna became aware of a large amount of rage and ferocity that she previously had not been in touch with or allowed herself to express.

As she moved the metaphor of "being the responsible adult ballerina" and then moved the metaphor of "being the carefree young girl who loved to dance," Joanna succeeded in gradually assimilating and synthesizing these polarized aspects of her self-experience. Through this movement process she discovered that she could combine the virtuosity that she had acquired over long years of study with the emotional spontaneity that she had known earlier as a carefree young girl. When some of her fellow performers commented that her dance performances now showed "some real spirit" and "spark," Joanna realized that she had undergone a profound physical, emotional, and behavioral self-transformation.

Joanna's splitting of what she considered to be her formal, responsible adult-self from her spontaneous childhood-self is reminiscent of the distinction that Winnicott (1980) drew between a person's "False Self" versus "True Self." He maintained that the "False Self" was a coping strategy developed by children to hide and protect their "True Self." He noted that the latter originated from the aliveness of the child's own body.

Phase Four: Termination

During phase four, clients begin to anticipate the end of the therapeutic relationship that they have forged over time with a "wise and caring other" as well as the end of the type of contact they have been able to forge over time with their own active imagination through a receptive and active movement process.

The loss of the therapeutic relationship and process are significant losses that must be mourned. For persons with issues of abandonment and separation this phase can be a particularly emotionally difficult one to negotiate. The loss of the therapeutic relationship is generally resolved when clients become convinced that its ending not only represents a significant personal loss but also a significant personal gain. That is, the loss of the therapeutic relationship attests to their having achieved a greater sense of self-mastery and the ability to forge more gratifying relationships with others that they care about.

RESEARCH-BASED EVIDENCE OF EFFECTIVENESS

A review of all DMT research studies published during 1974-1993 was conducted by Ritter and Low (1996). This review evaluated the efficacy of DMT with functioning as well as nonfunctioning adults and children, physically and mentally disabled individuals, elderly clients, and patients suffering from various kinds of physical illnesses. Initially the authors found a total of 95 research studies. When they applied the rigorous set of criteria they established as a standard for an adequate research design, only 23 studies met their criteria. The findings of these 23 studies can be summarized as follows: (1) positive changes in body attitude, self-acceptance and movement integration, lowered anxiety and lowered depression were found among noninstitutionalized adults, (2) modest positive effects with respect to movement and spatial awareness were manifested by developmentally disabled children, (3) improved body-image changes were revealed among adult arthritic patients, (4) improved motion and feelings of camaraderie were discovered among women suffering from breast cancer who were seen in DMT groups, and (5) increased capacity for independence, level of comfort with personal space, and degree of relaxation were found among individuals affected by traumatic brain injuries.

Unfortunately, Ritter and Low's (1996) DMT research review did not differentiate among research studies with respect to which type of DMT approach was used. Three studies which offer additional information with respect to the effects produced by short-term and long-term psychodynamic DMT groups found (1) significant increases in degree of self-actualization and body-self satisfaction among short-term psychodynamic DMT group participants; (2) positive changes in individual and interactive movement style among participants in long-term psychodynamic DMT groups and a shift in participants' perception of the therapist over time from "a container of participant's emotions" to "an interpreter of the meaning of participant's movement experience"; and (3) the emergence of four distinctive group movement patterns that appeared to reflect the ongoing psychodynamics of long-term psychodynamic DMT groups (Dosamantes-Alperson & Merill, 1980; Dosamantes, 1990, 1992). The findings of the last study offer empirical confirmation for the view that we continually and unconsciously move to shape and mold ourselves physically in response to the unfolding psychodynamics of our social-emotional environment.

Two broad issues that the DMT field needs to continue to address through further research are (1) the effectiveness of different DMT approaches with particular kinds of client populations and (2) the effectiveness and ethical concerns raised by the use of DMT with populations whose worldview differs widely from that of American DMT practitioners.

GUIDELINES FOR THE USE OF DMT

Persons who wish to obtain the theoretical and applied clinical training that is required to become an effective and ethical DMT practitioner have two options:

1. Pursue the MA degree in DMT from a graduate training program offered at one of several educational institutions in the United States that has received approval status from the American Dance Therapy Association. (A current list of such programs is available through the American Dance Therapy Association. Contact information about this professional organization is provided at the end of this chapter.)
2. Follow the alternative type of training that is outlined in the guidelines established by the ADTA. This second option is most suitable for those individuals who already possess a graduate degree in a related health care field and who are licensed as psychotherapists within their own state.

Psychotherapists who have no interest in pursuing the extensive training required to qualify as a registered dance therapist may still be able to benefit from their participation in DMT workshops or in DMT as a form of therapy for themselves. Such an exposure to DMT clinical work is likely to increase their sensitivity to the somatic, nonverbal dimensions of their clinical work.

One reason that extensive training is required to be an effective and ethical practitioner in this field is precisely because DMT is not about providing a prescribed set of mechanically performed exercises which can be repeated daily to achieve a pre-determined physical outcome or effect. In this respect, DMT is not like physical therapy.

Some characteristics that must always be taken into consideration when recommending DMT treatment to a client, include the personal and cultural history of the client, his or her emotional developmental level, chronological age, psychological strengths and weaknesses, and tolerance for regression. Clients such as John who have a difficult time regulating their emotional states and who undergo a maladaptive or structural regression that results in the experience of self-fragmentation are likely to require more structured kinds of movement experiences as well as a greater degree of emotional support and consistency from a dance therapist in order to achieve smaller kinds of physical and psychological changes than clients who function relatively well in the outside world, who can temporarily engage in a benign regressive process, and who are able to readily return to the world of consensually validated reality. The dance therapist who works with structurally regressed clients must be an experienced therapist who has worked with a wide variety of clients, does not fear becoming overwhelmed by the intensity of the altered states exhibited by clients who have become structurally regressed, and has moved through an in-depth psychodynamic therapeutic movement process herself.

In Western verbal psychotherapy, the areas of touch and physical contact with clients are highly taboo subjects and any physical intervention with clients tends to be cast automatically within the framework of some type of sexual intrusion on the part of the therapist. Generally verbal psychotherapists are admonished to refrain from having any physical contact with their clients for fear of being sued for some form of sexual harassment. The DMT field adopts a more neutral and differentiated stance toward the issue of "physical intervention" with clients. Most dance therapists would agree that a dance therapist must gauge any physical intervention (e.g., whether to mirror a client's movement or touch a particular client) in light of the particular client's emotional developmental level, the meaning such intervention would hold for the client, the benefit to be gained by the client, and the moment during the DMT treatment process when such an intervention would occur. Thus, when working with an autistic or mute client whose sole means of communicating with others is through his body and through body movement, many dance therapists would act to mirror the client's movement as a means of conveying to the client that he or she is emotionally attuned to the client's existential predicament.

Clinical Example

Even a seemingly harmless gesture such as the gentle patting of a client's back must be gauged by the dance therapist in light of a client's personal and cultural history, his or her psychological level of functioning, and when in the treatment process such physical contact occurs. The following clinical vignette underscores the importance of understanding what "being touched" means to a particular client during a particular moment of his treatment process. It illustrates how a well-intentioned DMT intern committed a clinical error that led to destructive consequences for the client:

> Following the end of a group DMT session conducted by her clinical supervisor, Carol, a young and inexperienced DMT intern gently patted a structurally regressed patient, Raymond, on his back (a gesture she considered to be a sign of support). Unfortunately, as soon as she did so, Raymond became unduly distraught, terrified, and immediately emotionally and cognitively decompensated. He kept repeating that he had "been poisoned" by her.
>
> What Carol failed to take into consideration was that Raymond, who had been psychiatrically diagnosed as a "paranoid schizophrenic patient," held a deep, delusional conviction that he would die if he were to be touched by another person.
>
> The training that DMT practitioners receive teaches them to consider the needs and emotional functional level of their clients and the psychodynamics of the ongoing treatment process. Dance therapists learn to time when a particular type of movement intervention might be appropriate and when not. For instance in the case cited above, perhaps at a later point in Raymond's DMT process, when he had already acquired a higher degree of trust in the DMT process and in Carol's capacity to contain his thoughts and emotions, he might have understood and appreciated her well-intentioned gesture of support.

In most psychodynamic DMT groups, the movement structure that is provided to participants during the initial phases of the DMT process is intended to acquaint group members with moving spontaneously in space, encourage their interactive movement dialogues with other group participants, and to create movement metaphors that provide a window to their symbolic inner life. Although the goals of all psychodynamic DMT approaches are dictated by a client's developmental, emotional, and physical needs, the duration of the therapeutic process often depends upon the treatment setting.

SHORT-TERM PSYCHODYNAMIC DMT

Short-term DMT is usually conducted within a group context in most institutional settings. Within institutional settings, the dance therapist provides a high degree of direction and concentrates on achieving several specific goals shared by most group members. The transference relationship is kept in the background, groups tend to be present-time oriented, and the date of termination is often determined in advance.

Clinical Example

During the 1980s I conducted a short-term DMT group with 14 male psychiatric patients who attended an outpatient psychiatric unit of a Veterans' Administration Hospital. The psychiatrist in charge of these patients' care described them as "impulsive and prone to drug addiction and violence." He recommended brief DMT for them so they could "achieve better control over their impulses and learn to become calmer." The group met for 10, two-hour long sessions. What follows is a description of the DMT process that unfolded in this group over a 10-week period:

> During early sessions, group participants were encouraged to become familiar and comfortable with their own body selves by focusing on the tension levels they found in various parts of their bodies and by learning to "let go" of the tension they experienced. Group members also learned to attend to the kinds of sensations and images that emanated from tense parts of their bodies. These kinds of movement experiences led one group member to spontaneously remark that he "got

the same kind of buzz by relaxing deeply as (he) did from drugs." Many in the group agreed with him. They seemed surprised to discover that they had the power to regulate the tension levels of their own bodies.

Participants then proceeded to get to know one another through movement. While standing in a circle facing each other, they began to explore sharing with one another "a movement that expressed how they felt in the moment." Then, they began to explore "trying on some one else's movement." At first group members took these experiences lightly and humorously. Over time, however, they became more seriously engaged in the movement process, and they expressed their appreciation about being able to get to know one another by "placing (themselves) in someone else's shoes." As the intimacy between group members increased, they simultaneously became increasingly anxious. Some mentioned that they "had not realized that (they) had been dancing with other men," an experience that many of them associated with "being gay."

I encouraged each participant to show the distance that he felt comfortable with when relating to another man as well as the kinds of movements that he felt comfortable with when relating to another man. Without exception, as each group member shortened the distance that he created between himself and another man, the movements that he engaged in assumed some combination of fighting qualities (e.g., pushing, shoving, elbowing, and kicking).

Following this experience I proceeded to work with the men in dyads. After selecting a partner who they felt comfortable moving with, I requested that they close their eyes and while sitting with their backs turned toward their partner begin to explore "giving and receiving each other's weight." As they did so, I introduced the notion of alternating between the movement qualities of "resisting" and "yielding." By sometimes resisting and sometimes yielding, the men began to connect with those aspects of themselves that they dreaded most, being vulnerable and expressing tenderness, aspects which they apparently equated with "being feminine." At the end of this movement experience many group participants allowed themselves to cry freely in each other's presence, without fearing being ridiculed or shamed by the other men in the group.

The male patients who participated in this short-term psychodynamic group were given an opportunity to experience themselves as the source of their own body tension. By learning to reduce the tension they found in various parts of their bodies, they also discovered a way to regulate their anxiety. This knowledge provided them with an alternative method for reducing their tension besides resorting to drugs. Group members also expanded their view of "what it means to be a man." They became open to the possibility that vulnerability and tenderness were not per se feminine emotional qualities.

LONG-TERM PSYCHODYNAMIC DMT

Long-term DMT is usually conducted within a private practice setting with individual clients. (This form of treatment is generally not reimbursed by health insurance companies.) In private open-ended individual DMT, the client generates and determines the movement themes that she or he will explore. The therapist systematically tracks the intersubjective relationship that unfolds between the client and him or her self over time. Sessions are past-time as well as present-time oriented and the termination date of therapy is open-ended. The case of Elizabeth illustrates the therapeutic process that unfolds in long-term psychodynamic individual DMT.

Clinical Example

I first met Elizabeth when she was in her early thirties and she was enrolled as a student in an introductory DMT group workshop at a local college. The workshop group met for a total of ten weeks twice weekly for two-hour long sessions each time. Workshop participants were provided with an open-ended movement structure that allowed them to become familiar with both active and receptive forms of movement. The movement structure provided sought to heighten each student's body-self awareness, to encourage participants' safe exploration of the environmental space through movement, to become engaged in movement interactions with others, and to generate movement metaphors that held special symbolic significance for them.

While Elizabeth attended all workshop sessions and participated fully during the movement part of the workshop sessions, she almost never commented upon her movement experience at the end of each session, a time that was always reserved by the therapist so that any group participant who wished could verbally share any aspect of his or her moved experience with others in the group. The only comment that she ever made was to say that she "enjoyed moving the images that she had visualized while lying down." I also noticed that whenever the group was engaged in a receptive movement exploration of their own internal symbolic experience, Elizabeth appeared to be deeply emotionally involved with whatever images she spontaneously generated from her own imagination. However, because she never spoke about her movement experience or the images that she had visualized, I could not fathom much about the content of these images nor the symbolic significance they held for her. Therefore, I was a bit surprised that when the movement workshop ended, she asked me whether I would be willing to consider working privately with her.

In individual long-term psychodynamic DMT work, the client is afforded an opportunity to obtain the full attention of the therapist and to set the direction, content, pace, and emotional tone of the DMT process, without having to take into consideration the needs and welfare of others, as is the case in most psychodynamic DMT groups. During her first DMT session, Elizabeth commented that she had enjoyed her workshop experience and mentioned liking the opportunity to have the "privacy" of moving alone without having to share her personal experience with others. She went on to say that she particularly liked those moments when she could "go inside" of herself and connect with her spontaneously emergent images "as though in a waking dream."

What follows is an outline of the various phases through which Elizabeth moved over the nearly two years that we worked together for hour-long sessions, twice a week.

Early Phases: Elizabeth Regresses and Returns
to an Early State of Isolation

During the early phases of our DMT work together, Elizabeth elected to spend several weeks being quiet and inwardly attentive to her own spontaneously emerging bodily sensations, kinesthetic and kinetic images. This time, however, her experience differed from her previous DMT workshop group experience in that she gradually began to verbally share the content of these images with me. In the therapeutic phases that followed, Elizabeth proceeded to transform these images into movement metaphors and verbal narratives that over time helped her bridge her internal symbolic life with significant aspects of her past and current relationships.

From the outset I became involved in tracking the somatic intersubjective relationship that evolved between us. For my part, I began to tune into my own bodily felt or somatic reactions as she moved and spoke (I have described the somatic intersubjective aspects of a therapist's experience in another publication, Dosamantes-Beaudry, 1997). Initially, I sensed that Elizabeth wanted to return to an earlier state of being, to a time when her emotional development had become derailed by some sort of trauma that she could not immediately recall or find the proper words to describe.

During the initial phase of the DMT process, Elizabeth seemed to be encapsulated within a cocoon of her own creation. After several weeks passed, I began to experience Elizabeth as though she were a neonate and also to sense that she had transformed me into a benign maternal figure whose primary psychological function was to watch over her and to see to it that no harm came to her. During this time, I observed Elizabeth becoming deeply involved in a world ruled by sensation and to be content to lie at the center of her well-protected sensual cocoon.

After some time elapsed, Elizabeth began to risk sharing and moving some of the images that she was visualizing. The images that emerged from her imagination provided me with a clue about the disruptive kinds of early relationships that had contributed to her creation of the encapsulated state in which she now found herself. One day, she shared the dream of having been given "a beautiful gift, a diamond necklace" by her mother but "instead of appreciating it and loving it (she) dreaded receiving it and experienced it as harmful." As she visualized her dream, she began to move receptively toward the diamond necklace and discovered that it was a "beautiful diamond choker." As she proceeded to place the diamond choker upon her neck, the necklace began to choke her and she found herself gasping for air and for her life, unable to breathe. When I asked her whether there was anything she could do to ease the pressure the necklace was exerting, she gasped and replied "no" and that she "felt totally helpless." However, she suddenly discovered that by releasing the clasp on the back of the necklace, she could breathe freely again.

Following this movement experience, Elizabeth began to recall that when she was an infant her mother had attempted to treat a serious chest congestion she had by covering her head with a towel and placing her over a pot of boiling water which exuded a vapor that was intended to clear up her congestion. Elizabeth experienced this event as "a terrifying one" because she felt "as though (her) mother was trying to suffocate (her)." To Elizabeth, her very depressed mother seemed to be emotionally unavailable to her. She also hated having to share her attention with a sister who was only a year younger than herself and sought to get her mother's attention by becoming ill. In therapy, Elizabeth reenacted her deep sense of maternal deprivation and abandonment with me by becoming ill with a cold prior to my first vacation leave. When I returned, she expressed a great deal of disappointment and rage over what she considered to be my "abandonment" of her.

Tustin (1990) claims that even persons who function relatively well in the outside world may be compelled to create an autistic type of auto-generated encapsulation when they prematurely experience a bodily separation from a nursing mother. The separation forces them to cope with intense feelings of emptiness, helplessness, and vulnerability with which they are not prepared to cope with effectively and instead experience as emotionally overwhelming. As a consequence, these children turn to their own bodily sensations as a source of comfort and protection. They create a psychological "auto-generated encapsulation" that protects them against the experience of an abrupt physical rupture from the mother and from further pain (Tustin, 1990, p. 117). According to Tustin, this is an extremely effective adaptation for shutting out the outside world and for being in control over whatever happens to one as an infant. She states:

> If the break in their continuation of "being" is occasioned by the trauma of an unduly harshness of bodily separateness is understood and worked over, the patient experiences a kind of psychic birth. (Tustin, 1990, p. 152)

Because I listened to the enraged accusations that Elizabeth leveled at me without retaliating in kind and helped her to perceive the connection that existed between her present experience of abandonment and her earlier experience of maternal abandonment, the therapeutic relationship survived her attacks and was not ruptured. Our transcendence of this critical emotional storm allowed Elizabeth to continue to experience the therapeutic relationship as a caring ambience that she found to be "soothing." She remarked that the therapeutic relationship stood in sharp contrast to the relationship that she once had with her own mother.

Elizabeth then began to explore the autistic, encapsulated world that she had created as a child through particular images that emerged from her dreams and fantasies. As she identified with each of these images through movement, she became aware of the painful toll her infantile autistic defense had exacted upon her as an adult.

Working Through Phase: Enacting the Beast Within
and Transcending Omnipotence, Rage, and Grandiosity

As Elizabeth became more familiar and trusting of the therapeutic environment, she began to move an aspect of herself that she often enacted with others in the outside world, but did not experience as ego dystonic. She rationalized what she considered to be her "feelings of superiority over others" by referring to her own "specialness." She considered herself to be a rather unique individual by virtue of her superior intellect as well as her ability to detect other peoples' motives by attending to their nonverbal behavior. She viewed this skill as "(her) own unique gift."

When Elizabeth spoke in this fashion, I felt as though she had become fused or merged with me and the therapeutic function that I was providing for her which she characterized as my "capacity to read other people's minds from their physical expressive behavior." By appropriating the same function that I served for her, she blurred any semblance of separation that might exist between us. By doing so, she transformed me into a self object that was under her control. The term self object refers to the supportive psychological function a therapist serves for a client who has not yet achieved a coherent and stable sense of self. Kohut (1984) coined the term "transmuting internalization" to refer to the process whereby clients appropriate particular psychological attributes modeled by their therapist in order to bolster their own tenuous sense of self and to function more effectively in the outside world (p. 99).

Elizabeth then began to enact her sense of entitlement and omnipotence through an identification that she formed and developed with a large black male bear that she had dreamt about (I took her identification with the black male bear of her dreams to be a manifestation of those aspects of herself that were instinctual or "shadow" aspects of her own self-experience that she could not consciously perceive). Jung (1968) referred to denied, unconscious aspects of a person's self that are projected onto other objects as a person's "shadow" (p. 174).

As Elizabeth transformed herself into the image of the black bear of her dreams, she stood upright and then began to walk on all fours ambling through the mountainous terrain that the bear considered to be his own. This bear could go anywhere that "he wanted to, and do anything he pleased." Then, the bear went through a deep "hibernation period" only "to wake up ravenously hungry" so he proceeded "to stuff himself full of blueberries until he felt he could burst." After he had had his fill he "decided to go into the town below and scare off some of the people that he encountered along the way, before they could take a pot shot at him with their rifles."

In Elizabeth's movement enactment of her dream fantasies, the bear's awakening from a period of hibernation seems to represent her desire for self-resurrection. The pride that she takes in her own self-sufficiency and the enormity and ravenousness of the bear's hunger reveal the strength of her oral deprivation. One can see that she protects herself against potential human harm by preempting potential external attacks through aggressive acts that have the intention of keeping any human who might harm her at bay.

Once Elizabeth gave vent to the bear's rage by demonstrating physically the many ways in which he could strike fear in others, the bear became a more passive, playful, and cuddly bear. He began to seek other animals that lived in the same mountain. He enjoyed playing games with other animals and allowed them to enter his turf without having to exact some form of retribution from them. As Elizabeth's rage subsided, she began to move beyond her own self-sufficient state to explore a world populated by others.

Elizabeth's enactment of her bear dream fantasies was followed by a physical identification with "a jolly green giant," who possessed more human-like qualities. When she physically transformed herself into this giant, she stood tall and made exaggerated large movements that allowed her to tower over anyone who came near her. However, unlike the black bear, this creature assumed a more playful human-like form and at times even showed some concern and empathy for the rest of the creatures that lived in the same town. In the outside world, Elizabeth began to exhibit some interest in interacting with other people.

While Elizabeth's fantasy of being a "jolly green giant" who got whatever he desired by overpowering others through his enormous size reflects a high level of narcissism, this giant, unlike the black bear character which had preceded it, was able to experience loneliness and to exhibit some form of concern for "the little people who lived in the town below."

Though Elizabeth still clung to her own sense of entitlement, she now seemed better able to manifest some interest and concern for the welfare of others. Her behavior in social settings outside of DMT sessions began to parallel her therapeutic experience. Elizabeth began to show an interest in socializing with other people and in dating members of the opposite sex. She no longer seemed to be so frightened of others nor so enraged by them. She was now able to put into words what previously she had only been able to express and to enact through imaginary self objects.

The nature of our intersubjective relationship also shifted dramatically. I experienced myself as gradually being transformed by her into a mother figure who could help her make sense of her imaginary movement experience through words and thereby increasingly help her build meaningful links between her inner symbolic world and her external interpersonal world.

Termination Phase: Taking Risks
and Planning for a Future

During the termination phase of her individual DMT sessions, Elizabeth reported becoming more interested in socializing with others outside of the DMT context. Apparently during this phase, she began to take the risk of dating men, which entailed making herself potentially vulnerable to rejection; something she dreaded because it forced her to reexperience the old wounds of her infantile depression. The fact that she was now willing to take the risk of rejection meant that she felt emotionally strong enough to handle whatever might transpire in her relationships with others.

She also began to make plans to continue her education. One day she announced that she had decided to become a psychologist and to make "use of (her) sensitivity to nonverbal experience in order to help others." Through this action, Elizabeth demonstrated that she had internalized those qualities that she had initially admired in the therapist and had developed an altruistic interest in helping others like herself who found themselves trapped in the same infantile autistic encapsulated state in which she had found refuge as a child.

The last time I saw Elizabeth was at a professional psychology conference where she informed me that she had indeed become a psychologist. She embraced me and expressed her gratitude for having "met (her) where she actually lived existentially" (referring to the infantile autogenic encapsulated state that she had been in when we first met).

CONCLUSION

DMT is a form of psychotherapy that makes use of body-movement as an instrument of consciousness to achieve body-mind integration and to promote self and group transformation. This contemporary Western body-based clinical practice challenges Euro-American culture's Cartesian view of the body. Unlike most verbal psychotherapies, DMT makes primary use of body movement as an instrument of consciousness. It differs from mechanistic "body therapies" in paying greater attention to the unfolding psychodynamics and to the derivation of the symbolic meaning clients generate from their own movement experience.

Short-term psychodynamic DMT tends to be conducted with groups in institutional settings, to be present-time oriented, and to be time-limited in nature. The goals and direction that the therapeutic process takes are generally predetermined by the professionals who are in charge of the clients' care. Long-term psychodynamic DMT tends to be conducted with individuals in a private practice setting. In long-term psychodynamic DMT, the client determines the content and the direction of the therapeutic process. The therapist systematically tracks the intersubjective relationship that unfolds between the client and herself. The process is open-ended in duration. In both short-term and long-term psychodynamic DMT, the dance therapist's primary concern is for the developmental, emotional, and physical welfare of his or her clients.

REFERENCES

Aalten, F. (1997). Performing the body, creating culture. In K. Davis (Ed.), *Embodied practices*. London: Sage Publications.

Bartenieff, I. (1972). Dance therapy: A new profession of a rediscovery of an ancient role of dance? *Scope, 7,* 6-18.

Bunney, J. (1980). Dance therapy: An overview. In R. Gibson (Ed.), *The use of the creative arts in therapy* (pp. 24-26). Washington, DC: American Psychiatric Association.

Davis, K. (1997). *Embodied practices*. London: Sage Publications.

Dosamantes, E. (1990). Movement and psychodynamic pattern changes in long term dance/movement therapy groups. *American Journal of Dance Therapy, 12*(1), 27-44.

Dosamantes, E. (1992). Spatial patterns associated with the separation-individuation process in adult long term psychodynamic movement therapy groups. *Arts in Psychotherapy Journal, 19,* 3-11.

Dosamantes, E. (1997). Reconfiguring identity. *Arts in Psychotherapy Journal, 24*(1), 51-57.

Dosamantes, E. (1998). Regression-reintegration: Central psychodynamic principle in rituals of transition. *Arts in Psychotherapy Journal, 25*(2), 79-84.

Dosamantes, E. (1999). A psychoanalytically-informed application of dance/movement therapy. In D.J. Wiener (Ed.), *Beyond talk therapy.* Washington, DC: American Psychological Association.

Dosamantes, E. (2001). The suppression and modern re-emergence of sacred feminine healing traditions. *Arts in Psychotherapy Journal, 28,* 31-37.

Dosamantes, E. (2003). *The arts in contemporary healing.* Westport, CT: Greenwood Publishing Group.

Dosamantes-Alperson, E. (1979). The intrapsychic and the interpersonal in movement psychotherapy. *American Journal of Dance Therapy, 3,* 20-31.

Dosamantes-Alperson, E. (1981). *Dance therapy: Psychiatric manual.* Columbia, MD: American Dance Therapy Association, Commission on Psychiatric Therapies.

Dosamantes-Alperson, E. & Merrill, N. (1980). Growth effects of experiential movement psychotherapy. *Psychotherapy: Theory, Research and Practice, 17*(1), 63-68.

Duggan, D., Bell, A., Orleans, F., Wexler, L., Bennett, R., & Greenberg, M. (1979). *Dance therapy.* Columbia, MD: American Dance Therapy Association.

Hanna, J.L. (1979). *To dance is human.* Austin: The University of Texas Press.

Jung, C.G. (1968). *Man and his symbols.* New York: Dell Publishing Group Inc.

Kohut, H. (1984). *How does analysis cure?* Chicago: University of Chicago Press.

Landy, D. (1997). Introduction to special issue on the state of the arts. *Arts in Psychotherapy Journal, 24*(1), 3-4.

Levy, F.J. (1988). *Dance/movement therapy: A healing art.* Reston, VA: American Alliance for Health Physical Education, Recreation and Dance.

Pallaro, P. (1995). Third European Therapies Conference. September 14-17, 1994, University of Ferrara, Italy. *American Journal of Dance Therapy, 17,* 141-144.

Ritter, M. & Low, K.G. (1996). Effects of dance/movement therapy: A meta analysis. *Arts in Psychotherapy Journal, 23,* 249-260.

Tustin, F. (1990). *The protective shell in children and adults.* London: H. Karnac Books Ltd.

Winnicott, D.W. (1980). *Playing and reality.* New York: Penguin Books.

Chapter 8

Music Therapy

Jennifer Jones

DEFINITION

According to the American Music Therapy Association (AMTA, 1999),

> Music therapists assess emotional well-being, physical health, social functioning, communication abilities, and cognitive skills through musical responses; design music sessions for individuals and groups based on client needs using music improvisation, receptive music listening, song writing, lyric discussion, music and imagery, music performance, and learning through music; participate in interdisciplinary treatment planning, ongoing evaluation, and follow up.

A definition by AMTA in 1997 cited in Davis, Gfeller, and Thaut (1999) defines music therapy as follows:

> (Music therapy) is the use of music in the accomplishment of therapeutic aims: the restoration, maintenance, and improvement of mental and physical health. It is the systematic application of music, as directed by the music therapist in a therapeutic environment, to bring about desirable changes in behavior. (p. 7)

Both descriptions cover the practice of music therapy with diverse clients ranging from infancy to old age and in need of treatment for

Introduction to Alternative and Complementary Therapies
© 2008 by The Haworth Press, Taylor & Francis Group. All rights reserved.
doi:10.1300/5987_08   *179*

a variety of conditions. The definition must accommodate music therapy with an infant in the ICU, a person in the final stages of Alzheimer's disease, a middle-aged woman with autism, and a college student with manic depressive illness.

Music therapists begin by assessing a client's needs and strengths, both through traditional methods of interviewing and observation and by documenting responses to music. Carefully selected music and music experiences are used to achieve the goals of therapy. The desired result of music therapy is similar to that of any other therapy—a change in behavior resulting in the improved welfare of the client. Techniques such as music and imagery, lyric discussion, and music improvisation are all potentially applicable in music therapy as psychotherapy. In addition, different types of music and diverse music experiences are potentially therapeutic. The music therapy process will be individualized for each person.

If one removes the references to music and music therapist in the above paragraphs, the protocol for treatment reads like the description of most forms of psychotherapy. Most treatment approaches involve assessment, treatment planning, and intervention with the client. However, the use of music *in* the therapeutic process and *as* the therapy is what distinguishes music therapy from other methods. A person's reactions to music are used in the assessment phase; treatment techniques involve music; and musical output (improvised music, written songs, songs selected by the client) is used in evaluating the effectiveness of the treatment. The board-certified music therapist is a trained musician who has studied music extensively, possesses a broad knowledge of styles and genres, and is capable of performing on several instruments and composing original music. Music therapists also study anatomy, psychology, and sociology. To say that the music therapist is a musician-turned-therapist would be inaccurate. Music therapy is an amalgam of music and therapy (Boxill, 1985). The effective music therapist must maintain a connection with each domain.

Scenario #1—Group Music Therapy in an Acute Psychiatric Hospital

The definitions and descriptions of music therapy give some clues as to what music therapists do and who they are. But how might a client react when offered music therapy? Consider the following scenario (Scenario #1). Imagine the experience of a patient in an acute unit of a psychiatric hospital or treatment center. A therapist enters the unit or ward and announces that it is time for music therapy. He or she invites the patients to come to the music therapy room for a session. Did he or she say *music* therapy? As a patient, what questions might come to mind when you hear the words *music therapy*? You might be wondering whether you have to "be musical" in order to join the group. You might wonder why music therapy is a part of the treatment plan at a psychiatric facility. You might wonder whether recordings of classical music will be played. You might wonder how music will help you get better.

These are logical responses from someone unfamiliar with music therapy in the treatment of mental health. It may seem out of place to have music as a therapy. Music is often associated with entertainment and leisure. Is the purpose of music therapy to provide entertainment? Perhaps the music therapist will perform for the group. What if you are supposed to perform? Performing music takes experience and practice. What if you do not play any musical instruments or have musical ability? Is there a reason to go to the music therapy group? What if music therapy means relaxing to classical music? Will it still work if you do not like classical music? If music therapy is just listening to music, you can do that alone. Why go to the music therapy group? What can a music therapist offer that you could not do for yourself?

Perhaps curiosity about music therapy convinces you to go with the therapist and other group members. The music therapist may explain some things about music therapy at the beginning of the session. She will likely tell the group that they do not need musical training to benefit from this group. It may be stated that while learning how to sing or play an instrument can have therapeutic value, the goal of this session does not include teaching musical skills. As you look around the room, this seems like a conflicting statement. There are drums of all sizes, guitars, pianos and keyboards, maracas and other shakers, a gong, xylophones, hand bells, and other instruments you cannot name. In addition to the instruments, there is a large collection of recorded music and songbooks. From the diversity and amount of equipment, it seems clear that more types of music than classical are a part of music therapy. There is also too much equipment for just the therapist to give a performance. A number of questions have been answered— music therapy is not a concert given by the therapist, is more than just relaxing to classical music, and does not require prior musical training.

The music equipment as described in Scenario #1 is a typical set-up for music therapy, including a variety of percussion instruments (drums, maracas, shakers, tambourines, bells, etc.), keyboards or pi-anos, guitars, and other instruments depending upon the therapist's skills and the needs of the clients. Collections of recorded music will be diverse, including instrumental and classical music, popular music (rock and roll, country, alternative rock, folk, rap, etc.), hymns and other religious music, jazz, and other genres. Songbooks and collec-tions of sheet music will be equally diverse. Music therapy sessions may take place in a room set up with the equipment, or the therapist may bring the equipment to the group. In addition to inpatient hospi-tals, music therapists work in other mental health settings, including day treatment and outpatient centers, substance abuse programs, forensic units, and in private clinics. Music therapists work with chil-dren, adolescents, adults, and those over 65. Music therapy may be provided individually, in a group, or as a part of family therapy. It may be included in interdisciplinary treatment, through referral of a treating physician or therapist, or may be sought out as a primary therapy by the patient or caregiver.

Let us continue with the music therapy session at the psychiatric hospital. The session described will incorporate techniques common to most music therapy practices, but it is important to keep in mind that music therapy is a highly flexible process in which no two thera-pists are alike and no two sessions are identical. A group of eight people is assembled in a room filled with musical instruments and re-cordings. As the group enters, a song is playing. The new members of the group ask about the song. The music therapist states it is a song chosen in a previous session. The song playing is "Desperado" by the Eagles. The music therapist lets the returning group members explain why the song was chosen to open this session. The therapist allows for comments about what the song now means.

The music therapist observes the discussion and realizes that only the returning group members are sharing their thoughts. He or she se-lects a music experience that will allow each member an opportunity to express feelings and open up interaction among the new members and returning members. He or she explains that the group is going to have an opportunity to express themselves through playing music with drums. He or she tells the group how to play each of the different types of drums, either by using their hands or with sticks called mallets. He or she directs the group to repeat after him or her the rhythm he or she played. Some group members watch carefully in order to play the rhythm while others listen and repeat the rhythm. She observes that some group members struggle on complicated patterns, some play boldly while others are timid, but most members of the group are successful in imitating her rhythms.

Using her observations of the rhythmic imitation task just completed, the music therapist selects a rhythmic pattern for the group to play together, taking into consideration the level of complexity needed for success. The group repeats a pattern of playing for eight beats followed by eight beats of silence. Once the group has mastered the pattern, the therapist explains to the group that in the silence, each person may play anything he or she wishes to express. At the end of each person's music, the group will play the eight beats together. After each person has played, the therapist asks if any of the group have expressed similar thoughts in their music. Once the musical similarities are discussed, the music therapist instructs those who played similar music to gather into small groups and talk about what they expressed. She facilitates the conversations. The small groups return and share the experience. Some groups express similar emotions while other groups find they did not express the same thoughts or emotions. The music therapist guides the discussion about expressing emotions and being understood by others. Depending upon the client's needs and readiness, the music therapist guides individuals to discuss the present musical experience, emotions resulting from the experience, or relate the emotions and experiences to personal life choices.

The music therapist quickly analyzes the content of the dialogue in order to select a final song to close the therapy session. In conjunction with the musical preferences of the group members, the music therapist selects a song that supports the discussion on emotion and understanding. The song chosen is "Sunshine on My Shoulders" by John Denver. He or she instructs the group to let the song help them to continue their reflections on their emotions. The therapist sings the song and plays the guitar for accompaniment. Some of the group members know the song and sing along, while others actively listen. The music therapist listens to brief closing comments and reminds the group that this song will start the next session. He or she encourages the group members to reflect on the song and the emotions experienced in the music therapy session. The group members leave the music therapy room and return to the unit.

The Music Therapy Process in Scenario #1

In the previously described scenario, the music therapist chose the music and music experiences to achieve the goals and objectives for treatment. The goals of the therapist included recalling the progress of the last session, establishing a nonthreatening rapport, increasing group cohesion, assessing psychomotor functioning and concentration, providing for self-expression, and supporting the emotional needs of the group members. The music experiences included recorded music, improvised music performed by the group members, and a song performed by the therapist. The session also included verbal dialogue about the music, the experience of performing/playing music, and expression of emotions. The techniques discussed are commonly used by music therapists, though a number of other techniques, songs, or music experiences could have been equally successful. Part of music therapy's effectiveness lies in its flexibility and adaptability.

The music therapy session began with a song playing as the group entered. The song established that music would be the focus of the treatment session. It prompted previous group members to recall the last session and provided opportunities for a nonthreatening dialogue about the music. As the music therapist assessed the need for group members to interact with each other more, the music intervention changed from listening to drumming. Creating music together integrated former and new group members. The improvised music provided common ground and formed the basis for small group discussion. The improvised music and subsequent discussions provided the therapist with another opportunity for intervention and allowed for a deeper exploration of emotions and thoughts. The music therapist chose to conclude the session with a song, which served as a transition for the next session, allowing for some continuity in the group process despite the entrance and exit of group members.

While the music used for music therapy is carefully selected, the process is in no way scripted. When selecting music for treatment, the effective music therapist considers the many elements of music (harmony, rhythm, timber, instrument selection, as well as others), the brain's responses to music, the client's music preferences and past experiences, the needs for developing therapeutic rapport and group cohesion, and the available musical resources. An accurate selection of music may facilitate the expression of inarticulate thoughts (Draper, 2001), arouse feelings and imagery (Halpern & Savary, 1985), provide a safe, confrontive tool (Clendenon-Wallen, 1991), and elicit changes in affect (Goldstein, 1990; Thaut 1989).

HISTORY OF MUSIC THERAPY

The roots of modern-day music therapy are in the psychiatric programs of United States' Veteran's hospitals developed during the 1940s (Peters, 2000). In a recent survey of music therapists, the mental health field continues to be the largest single category of populations served by music therapists, and represents 21 percent of the respondents (AMTA, 2003, p. 213). Though the professional organization of music therapists was established in the United States in 1950 (Peters, 2000), the use of music for healing is centuries old. Music is found in cultures throughout the world, from the most primitive to the current level of civilization. Jourdain (1997) concludes that music must come fairly easily for most humans.

Centuries ago, a person suffering symptoms of mental illness or emotional distress was often considered to be possessed by an evil spirit. Health and disease were associated with supernatural forces, as was music (Davis, Gfeller, & Thaut, 1999). A healer used music to connect with the supernatural and bring about healing. The shaman, also known as a witch doctor or medicine man, has been found in a number of cultures, including Native American and African cultures (Peters, 2000). The shaman used drumming, chanting, singing, and other instruments, such as bells and rattles, and elaborate costumes in the healing rituals. Though the specific practices in music and healing used by the shaman varied from group to group, the purpose of the music was often to induce a trance-like state in the afflicted person (Winn, Crowe, & Moreno, 1989). This state of altered consciousness was achieved by listening to repetitive drumming or chanting. The shaman's music was also intended to contact the spirit world and was used to bring forth dreams, songs, and imagery from what is now recognized as the unconscious (Alvin, 1975; Peters, 2000). Winn (Winn, Crowe, & Moreno, 1989) describes the process in the following manner:

> To the shaman, the act of therapy involves going beyond the seen reality of consciousness and into another level of awareness, known in shamanic traditions as the spirit world, in order to bring back information regarding the patient's loss of personal power that has allowed the disease. (p. 67)

The Greeks strongly influenced the role of music in society and in healing. According to the Greeks, music could "heal sickness, purify the body and mind, and work miracles in the realm of nature" (Grout & Palisca, 1988, p. 3). The Greek God Apollo was the God of Music and the God of Medicine, perhaps signifying the connection of music to healing. Disease was a result of "disharmony" and music could restore this state of harmony (Peters, 2000). Peters (2000) wrote, "Since the Greeks found that different types of music and different modes had fairly predictable effects on human conduct and emotions, they began to apply music systematically as both curative and preventative medicine" (p. 22). Christian beliefs in the Middle Ages conflicted with Greek beliefs about the cause of disease. Physical ailments were seen as punishment for sins, and mental illness was caused by possession by evil (Davis, Gfeller, & Thaut, 1999). Hymns were sung to saints who could provide protection against illness (Peters, 2000). Despite the differing assumptions as to the cause of disease, both the Christians and the Greeks influenced practices that called for the use of *specific* music in healing.

The nineteenth century is notable in the development of music therapy. As music composition flourished during the Baroque (1600-1750) and Classical periods (1750-1820) (Grout & Palisca, 1988), skilled musicians increased in number and availability. One major development in the history of music therapy occurred in London in the summer of 1891 when Frederick Harford established the Guild of

St. Cecilia (Davis, 1989). The Guild organized a group of "on-call" musicians to provide live music for patients in hospitals. Medical practices at the time were primitive and often resulted in death. Music as therapy was a much more appealing alternative to treatments such as bloodletting. Lacking any psychiatric medications, a common treatment for mental illness was for the patient to sleep. The technique employed was "to help patients focus attention toward the music which would lull them to sleep" (Davis, 1989, p. 19). This type of music therapy was reported in British medical and music journals of the time.

Published articles advocating and explaining the use of music as therapy in the treatment of mental illness and emotional distress appeared during the same century in the United States. In 1804 and 1806, dissertations written by two medical students, Edwin Atlee and Samuel Matthews, at the University of Pennsylvania discussed the effects of music on emotion and mood. Atlee reportedly instructed one patient to resume playing the flute as a part of treatment (Davis, Gfeller, & Thaut, 1999). Matthews recommended that the therapist match the mood of the client with music and gradually modify the music to change the client's mood (Peters, 2000). Musicians were hired in New York City to perform for mental patients at Blackwell Island (Davis, Gfeller, & Thaut, 1999) and Utica State Hospital (Peters, 2000). Neurologist James Leonard Corning researched music and imagery during dream states in hopes of finding ways to transfer pleasant images and emotions into waking hours (Peters, 2000). The late nineteenth century witnessed collaboration between musicians and physicians. The responses to music from anecdotal and controlled studies were documented and published. The primary treatment technique involved the patient listening to music, usually performed live by local musicians and sometimes supervised by a therapist or physician.

In the twentieth century, research on music's effects on the mind and body continued. Techniques and training in music therapy advanced with the first organizations and courses in music therapy. Four women were particularly influential in developing the specific use of music for therapy. Eva Vescelius was a trained singer who performed in hospitals and asylums. She developed a course for musicians, established a professional organization for music therapy in 1903, and published a short-lived journal, titled *Music and Health*

(Davis, Gfeller, & Thaut, 1999; Peters, 2000). Isa Maud Ilsen, a musician and nurse, and Margaret Anderton, a pianist, both worked with veterans of World War I. They taught courses in music therapy at Columbia University in New York and advocated for hospital musicians to have training prior to working with patients. Ilsen, like Vescelius, established a professional organization in 1926, the National Association for Music in Hospitals (Davis, Gfeller, & Thaut, 1999). Prior to her death in 1944, Harriet Ayer Seymour, a well-trained musician and one-time piano teacher at the Julliard School of Music in New York City, penned the first handbook of music therapy (Davis, 1996). She claimed to have trained 500 "musical doctors" in her career (Davis, 1996, p. 35). Her techniques involved a group of musicians playing for patients under the guidance of a music therapist. The client was given a word or phrase to repeat to him or her self as the musicians performed.

Music therapists working in the 1940s in Veterans Administration hospitals and state mental hospitals were mostly volunteer musicians. As the demand for music therapy increased with return of soldiers from World War II, a demand for training brought about the first college degree in music therapy offered at what is now Michigan State University in 1944 (Peters, 2000). Other universities soon commenced training, and degrees were offered at the University of Kansas, Chicago Music College, and College of the Pacific (Davis, Gfeller, & Thaut, 1999). Collegiate training largely focused on the uses of music therapy with the mentally ill, as most music therapists treated this population.

The short-lived professional organizations created in the early part of the twentieth century were replaced by the National Association for Music Therapy, established in 1950 during the Music Teachers National Association annual meeting in New York City. The National Association for Music Therapy (NAMT) was formed from the committee on music therapy, a group that was originally part of the music teacher's association. In 1971, a second music therapy association, the American Association for Music Therapy, or AAMT, served music therapists predominantly in the New York and New England areas. In 1998, the two associations, NAMT and AAMT, united to form the American Music Therapy Association, or AMTA—the association that now governs the profession. As the number of trained music therapists increased, a need was recognized for professional certi-fication. The Certification Board for Music Therapists was established in 1983 (Certification Board for Music Therapists, 2003). Since 1986 it has been fully accredited by the National Commission for Certifying Agencies (NCCA), and nearly 4,000 music therapists have attained the MT-BC credential (Certification Board for Music Therapists, 2003).

Early practitioners of music therapy were as varied as shamans, priests, physicians, and volunteer musicians. Today's music thera-pists are trained in collegiate programs culminating in bachelor's de-grees or their equivalents. The mastery of music and competency as a musician dominate the training of a music therapist. The study of mu-sic foundations accounts for 45 percent of the bachelor's degree in music therapy (American Music Therapy Association, 2001).

In addition to music study, the degree includes an internship of 900-1,040 hours of supervised clinical training. Following degree completion, music therapists take a national certification examina-tion. Applicants who pass the exam are awarded the credential MT-BC, or are music therapist board certified. One hundred continuing education credits must be completed every five years to maintain the credential (MT-BC). Music therapy's clinical validity is recognized by the Health Care Financing Administration (HCFA), the Joint Commission on the Accreditation of Health Care Organizations (JCAHO), the Rehabilitation Accreditation Commission (CARF), and the National Rehabilitation Caucus (NRC) (AMTA, 1999, p. 9).

WHY MUSIC?

Music possesses many qualities that make its use as a psycho-therapeutic technique quite appropriate. Music is highly accessible in our current society. We can listen to music from recordings, select music from numerous radio stations, or attend live performances. Music can be easily created or re-created by singing, humming, drum-ming, or playing other instruments. Most people on a daily basis en-gage in one of these musical activities. We are exposed to music in our daily situations. At sports events, we hear music that may increase our sense of loyalty for the "home" team or coordinate our behavior for a cheer. Commercially, music is used to identify products (jingles), encourage consumers to stay longer in stores to buy more merchandise

(MuZak), and to stay "on-hold" on the telephone longer (Radocy & Boyle, 1979). Music is used to commemorate holidays and recognize special events, such as graduation ceremonies, weddings, and so on. We are exposed to or we choose different kinds of music at different times in our lives—lullabies as children, rebellious music in our teens, and love songs in our young adult years.

In their own lives, most people have used music to change behaviors, moods, emotions, and situations. Consider the following example. After a difficult day at work, you get into your car for the commute home. The music playing on the radio station seems instantly irritating to your already stressed mood. Perhaps you change the station several times and finally find the perfect music. Your tension decreases, and you experience a sense of calm. Most of us recognize when we have found the right music for our commute just as easily as we recognize the wrong music.

Consider another example. You are caring for a nine-month-old child whose parent has just left to go shopping. The child is crying despite your comforting words and seems inconsolable. You sing to the child and rock her to the rhythm of your song. She turns to watch your face, listens carefully, and stops crying. The choice to sing to the crying child seems nearly instinctual. Music clearly influences our moods and behaviors. What music would your choose for a romantic dinner for two? What music would motivate you to complete chores? You likely would choose different selections to elicit different responses.

The properties of music, the brain's response to music, a person's associations with music, and the experience of music in a therapeutic relationship are elements that make music therapy a unique form of psychotherapy. To the physicist, music is merely sound created by vibrations traveling through the medium of air. The definition of music as simply a series of vibrations may seem stark, but the vibrations experienced through music make it a multisensory event. In fact, the human body absorbs up to two-thirds of the sounds striking it (Jourdain, 1997), a factor significant not only to music therapists, but also to professionals who design auditoriums and concert halls. Sound not only enters the ears to be processed by the brain, but it is also experienced by the entire body. This experience of sound can be particularly intense in the presence of live performers. (Remember the shaman's day-long drumming.)

Is sound synonymous with music? Crashing ocean waves create sound. Worn brake pads create sound. Wind chimes create sound. These sounds are not generally called music. Titon and Slobin (2002) define music as "meaningfully organized sound" (p. 17). Music is organized in a number of ways. Music is ordered in time, known as rhythm. Nature is time-ordered; consider the change of seasons or lunar cycles as examples. The human body is dependent upon rhythm, as is evident in the heartbeat, respiration, and gait. The rhythm of music often prompts movement, a tapping foot, swaying hips, and activated muscles (Davis, Gfeller, & Thaut, 1999). The brain is awakened by rhythm, also called pulse. Jourdain (1997) wrote, "Psychologically, pulse constitutes a renewal of perception, a reestablishment of attention. It is a basic property of our nervous system that they soon cease to perceive phenomena that do not change" (p. 126). The rhythm of music assists in maintaining active attention. The subtle, constant changes in music's rhythmic structure renew our attention. Music is also organized into melodies and harmonies. Farnsworth (1969) offered, "Music is composed of patterns of sound acceptable to the people of some culture" (p. 17). Each culture defines when a collection of pitches across time establishes a melody and is called music. People in China construct melodies differently from people in India or Indiana. Still, most people can recognize what is music, even if it comes from a different culture.

Music scholars, psychologists, and philosophers have long debated a clear definition of music. The challenge for music therapists is to accept a definition that is broad enough to cover the range of music experiences used in therapy. Consider the shaman's day-long drumming. Was this music? What about the drumming in scenario #1? The shaman's musical ability would have been obvious. His musical output would have evidenced his experience and training. The drumming created in the music therapy session by people seeking treatment would haven been considerably less proficient. Players could have been "off-beat," could have played too few beats or too many, or the group could have failed to begin playing on time. Was it still music? Is music defined by proficient production or by intention and effort? Music therapists consider these factors when defining music. Bruscia (1998) clarifies perhaps the most relevant factor for music therapists for determining what music is. He wrote, "Music therapy operates on the assumption that music experience is meaningful to clients, and that clients can use music to make meaningful changes in their lives" (p. 94).

The word "meaning" appears in more than one definition of music. The organized sounds must have meaning to the entire culture to be considered music, and a music therapist counts on music having meaning to individuals in therapy. Much of the way we assign meaning is through experience. Music is present in our lives from infancy to the grave. Jourdain (1997) wrote, "Something has meaning when it somehow represents our experience of the world or of ourselves" (p. 272). Music has meaning when it conveys something to us, and when we feel we can relate to it. Once meaning is assigned to music, a form of communication has taken place, an understanding between beings.

Music is often described as a language, specifically as a language of the emotions (Farnsworth, 1969). Draper (2001) describes music as being able to give expression to inarticulate thoughts and feelings. In music therapy, the client can express himself through making music, assign meaning to music while listening to music, and communicate nonverbally with the therapist. When personal emotions are too intense to verbalize in therapy, music can be a less threatening alternative. People in therapy are often seeking a way to express themselves or at other times are seeking to feel understood. Music therapy can accommodate both needs, often simultaneously. Music conveys a connection to human emotions in general while respecting each person's unique experiences. The "nonspecificity of the emotions elicited" (Halpern & Savary, 1985, p. 94) opens the possibilities of music to provide access to any type of emotion. Though music may not consistently inspire a specific emotion in a listener, it resonates with emotions and can bring to that listener a greater awareness of specific emotions.

Not only can music be used to express emotions, it can also stimulate emotion and change emotional/affective states in the listener (Goldstein, 1990; Thaut, 1989). Examples of this are abundant in the film industry. Music is used to induce fear during horror films, intensify sadness in dramas as the main character dies, or produce feelings of happiness when love conquers all. This is not to say that a selection of music will produce the same mood or emotion in all people under any given circumstance. In the example of music that accompanies a film, the condition is the same—people watching a movie and generally expecting to be entertained. Little psychological harm is caused if the musical score fails to heighten the moviegoer's experience.

Clearly more caution is warranted when using selected music for music therapy within a psychotherapy session. Generally, music therapists begin by matching the music to the client's starting mood state, a technique known as the iso principle (Peters, 2000). Both Farnsworth (1969) and Thaut (1989) acknowledge that a listener's starting mood, cultural experiences, and need for stimulation will affect the mood response to music. Halpern and Savary (1985) recognized that most traditional music is based on cycles of tension and release. This sense of tension and release is created through the organization of music by its rhythm, harmony, and melody. Halpern and Savary (1985) continue that this tension and release in music is "exciting to the emotions . . . helpful in generating imagery that the therapist may use in psychotherapy" (p. 143). Music mimics our emotional experiences (Jourdain, 1997).

Bruscia (1998) clarifies that music used in psychotherapy is not intended to necessarily placate the client. He wrote, "When the goal is psychotherapeutic, the client is engaged in music experiences that evoke the feelings and interpersonal dynamics that are problematic, while also experiencing their resolution or transformation through the music" (pp. 107-108). Music therapists use music at times to bring about emotional conflict and release through music experiences. Nolan (1989) discussed the music therapy treatment of Tina, a 25-year-old woman recovering from bulimia. He stated that she had perfectionistic tendencies and ambivalence toward her father and male relationships. Tina was in group music therapy session using musical improvisation. She frequently chose higher pitched instruments and avoided lower tones calling them "guys." The music therapist encouraged her to explore the lower tones as the group played with her for support. Tina began crying during the music and expressed tension through her affect. The music experience provided an opportunity for these painful emotions to surface in a controlled, safe, supportive environment. Tina told the music therapist that prior to this experience "she had not been able to cry for more than a few seconds without resorting to food" (Nolan, 1989, p. 50).

Music's emotional nature is clear, as is its purposefulness for accessing the emotions in psychotherapy. Creating music through improvisation allows the client to make many choices about how to express emotion. Listening to certain selections of music can influence mood, but not in a prescriptive manner. Farnsworth (1969) acknowledged that musical compositions could be placed into mood categories but "will not invariably arouse the moods in terms of which they have been described" (p. 79). One cannot simply choose a piece of music categorized as happy and play it for a depressed person and expect a cure. Peters (2000) wrote,

> While some general effects of music with certain characteristics that will be true for many people may be predicted, it is important to remember that how any particular individual will react to a particular piece of music is determined to a large extent by that individual's previous experience with music. (p. 53)

Bruscia (1998), too, acknowledges the personal experience of listening to music and speaks further to its use in psychotherapy. He states,

> Thus, the way a person makes or listens to music is a direct manifestation of that person's unique identity as a human being, reflecting not only who the person is but also how he or she deals with various situations. (p. 140)

The responses to music displayed by clients are a reflection of the clients themselves. The music therapist has employed music to illicit these responses.

Music therapists *use* music, and the music is a means to an end—which is to discover the emotional life and coping strategies of the client. Music does not function "passively as a medicine, but requires that the patient participate" (Jourdain, 1997, p. 302). The person in therapy must be open to the experience and must be a willing participant. The music in music therapy will act "almost as a co-therapist by evoking emotional responses . . . in ways not open to the human therapist, who is limited to words" (Halpern & Savary, 1985, p. 102). The relationships established in music therapy are triadic and consist of the music itself, the client, and the therapist (Peters, 2000). The nonverbal nature of music and its emotional connection allow for the client to "work" on emotion without verbal processing. MacKay (2002) writes, "The emotional, expressive nature of music can serve as a bridge to self-awareness, insight, and identification of feelings. Music stimulates association, affect, and imagery in ways that analytical, verbal process cannot" (Paragraph 1). Nolan (1989) wrote,

> Although the discussion can assist in concretizing the client's awareness of feeling associations, interpersonal role, and reality testing, extensive talking at this time (following music improvisation) can create a shift from the feeling state brought on by the musical interplay to a more restricted intellectualized defensive state. (p. 50)

In addition to unique personal experiences possible with music, music is a highly social phenomenon. The examples given in the text of sports events, weddings, religious ceremonies, and holiday celebrations support the social uses of music. Alvin (1975) calls music the "most social of all arts" which has "affected the man involved in it either as a participant or as a spectator" (p. 88). Humans are accustomed to experiencing music in groups. The concert performed for a crowd of thousands is an example of the group musical experience. It is rare for a musician to choose to perform only for him or her self throughout his entire existence.

Group experiences in music therapy begin with the common ground of group members having experienced music socially with others. Music can be familiar and is usually comfortable. As group music experiences unfold, interpersonal interaction becomes necessary. Individuals can begin to recognize their patterns of interaction, whether constructive or destructive (Davis, Gfeller, & Thaut, 1999). People seeking therapy often feel isolated and alone in their experience. Music therapy offers a "shared vulnerability" (Richards & Davies, 2002, p. 22) through the mutual experience of music. Plach (1980) states that music in a group therapy session provides a common and dependable starting place for discussion and personal work. In the music therapy scenario #1, the song was selected by the group as a "theme" song—one that reflected the emotions, opinions, and experiences of the group at that time. The song was again played at the beginning of the next session to "reorient" the group to the established identity, and to bring them back together as a unit. During the drumming in scenario #1, the group had to act cooperatively in order to achieve success. Each person had to listen and wait for his or her turn and play with the entire group. Interdependence was necessary for the music to be successful. Interpersonal relationships were further explored as the small groups gathered to discuss the music produced. The music therapy process described in scenario #1 allowed for group experiences that provided both challenge and success in relating to others.

In summary, music therapists use music for the unique qualities that it offers. First, it is a sensory experience, stimulating muscles and the sense of hearing, creating felt vibrations, and, in live music, providing a visual component. For a client who is understimulated or in a sterile environment, such as a psychiatric facility, music can provide welcome sensations for the body. Second, despite the challenges in defining music, it is an organized, meaningful experience for humans. It stimulates attention and resonates with our life experiences, both personally and culturally. It provides a language system for emotions. It stimulates emotions in listeners and within a therapeutic framework can aid in identifying and expressing distressing emotions. Music is both a group and a personal experience, making it suitable for group therapy and individual therapy. Music is used like a carefully crafted tool to bring about change. It can be an object, a symbol, a language, and a group experience, while remaining uniquely personal to each listener.

MUSIC THERAPY TECHNIQUES

Music therapy techniques used in psychotherapy are individualized for clients. The client can listen to music, perform music, create music, discuss music, relax to music, participate in guided imagery in music (GIM), or use music recreationally. Music therapists employ a variety of styles and types of music in their work and use music in a variety of ways to bring about therapeutic change for clients. The music used in these techniques can be performed by the therapist, by clients, or may be from recordings. Any given music therapy session could utilize only one or a combination of music experiences. Music therapy supports the diverse needs of people at different levels of functioning and is responsive to individual needs and capabilities. The techniques used in music therapy are also adapted to accommodate various treatment modalities and psychological theories. While there is no script or "cookbook" of music therapy techniques, the following techniques are loosely categorized.

Individual or Group Music Therapy

Following a careful assessment of the client, the music therapist must consider if group or individual music therapy will best meet that person's needs. Peters (2000) and Hanser (1987) acknowledge that often a facility's structure and financial limitations determine the setting for therapy, as group treatment is believed to be more cost effective than individual therapy. Both group and individual music therapy offer the client unique experiences, fiscal considerations notwithstanding. The individual music therapy session provides a one-to-one relationship. Peters (2000) states that the individual session "provides unique opportunities for initial explorations of a client's individual skills, preferences, and problems" (p. 72). Group therapy provides experiences with a peer group allowing for the exchange of feedback capitalizing on the social nature of music and allowing clients to observe different models of behavior. Even within a group therapy setting, individual needs can be addressed.

The success of group music therapy has been documented in inpatient treatment for substance abuse (Dougherty, 1984; James & Freed, 1989; Murphy, 1983), inpatient therapy with children (Friedlander, 1994), inpatient therapy for adults with mental illness (Butler, 1966; James & Freed, 1989), treatment for posttraumatic stress disorders through GIM (see later section) (Blake & Bishop, 1994), inpatient treatment for eating disorders (Hilliard, 2001a; Justice, 1994), outpatient substance abuse programs (Treder-Wolff, 1990), and school-based group bereavement therapy for children (Hilliard, 2001b). Group music therapy sessions can provide the therapist with a wealth of information about clients. The client's interaction with the music, the therapist, and other group members provides much needed assessment information. The client's ability to express emotions, respond to feedback, and interact successfully with others will cue the therapist to either continue group music therapy or refer the client for individual music therapy sessions. Group music therapy can decrease isolation (Murphy, 1983), increase interpersonal awareness since group music making requires interdependence, and contribute to the development of significant interpersonal relationships (Rio & Tenney, 2002).

Included in the documented successes in individual music therapy sessions are the treatment of a woman with schizo-affective disorder (Dvorkin, 1982), a 12-year-old boy with low self-esteem and a conduct disorder diagnosis (Kivland, 1986), an adult man with generalized anxiety disorder (Tyson, 1987), an elderly prison-patient with Alzheimer's disease (Vaughn, 1993), a woman with loss issues (Warja, 1994), an adult woman with a history of childhood abuse (Ventre, 1994), and individuals with schizophrenia (Pavlicevic, Trevarthen, & Duncan, 1994). A client who is unable to contribute to group music experiences or has limited verbal interaction may benefit from the intensity of a one-on-one relationship. The music therapist may be better able to meet the client at his or her functioning level more easily in an individual setting than in a group situation.

Often, clients with a musical background are referred for individual music therapy (Dvorkin, 1982; Tyson, 1987). As previously stated in this chapter, musical ability is not necessary for participation in music therapy, but clients with a high degree of musical skills allow the music therapist to demand more musically from the client. Tyson (1987) reported on the individual music therapy with Andrew, a violist who was concurrently in psychoanalysis. The music therapy techniques included music instruction in breathing, posture, voice and singing instruction, along with coaching Andrew in performing on his viola. Andrew's "psychological conflicts were sharply projected into the sphere of music" (Tyson, 1987, p. 54). Tyson (1987) wrote that, "The groundwork for resolution lay in the analysis of body movement utilized by the patient in singing and instrumental performance" (p. 55). His musical ability allowed the therapeutic process to evolve out of body movements evincing his anxiety, lack of self-confidence, and disrupted body image.

Dvorkin (1982) published a case study of a 26-year-old woman initially diagnosed with schizophrenia and major affective disorder. The woman, called M. in the report, showed little interest during group music therapy at an inpatient facility, but repeatedly asked to play the piano. M.'s piano skill (able to play simple pieces, relative ease at the piano) was likely the result of piano lessons, though she offered the music therapist no history of her music training. Over the eight months of treatment reported in the case study, M. was able to produce music to express negative emotions. She found ways to problem solve in her created piano improvisations that she initially disliked, instead of abandoning the music altogether, as it was her tendency to avoid con-flict. M. played music on the piano that was labeled "safe" by the therapist, and M. performed this music after confronting difficult emotions. The final stages of the music therapy included in the report reflect efforts to connect M.'s music to her affect. Similar to An-drew's therapy, M.'s piano improvisation allowed the manifestation of psychological symptoms that were addressed through demanding musical tasks.

Some music therapy techniques and psychological models are based specifically on individual therapy approaches. The Bonny meth-od of GIM was developed as an individual music therapy technique (Bonny, 1994), and is now also used in group situations. Analytically based music therapy through improvisation may be an individual music therapy approach, as was the case report of Andrew (Tyson, 1987). Music-assisted relaxation, particularly within a systematic de-sensitization framework, may be used in individual music therapy. Most music therapy techniques can easily be adapted for group or individual music therapy.

Active Listening–Based Techniques

Therapist-Selected Music

Because of its familiarity to most individuals, listening to music places minimal demand upon the client. In order to receive maximum benefit of the music listening experience, the client must be open to the experience and use the opportunity provided by the therapist. Mu-sic selected for a listening experience may be instrumental music or popular music. The music therapist probably cues the listener to be attentive to the music, as the music is not intended to be "background" but to play an active role in the process.

The music is chosen to generate specific responses. The desired responses may be pleasant or unpleasant sensations, thoughts, or emotions. In group settings, more than one opinion, experience, or emotional reaction is likely. Plach (1980) states, "Music is a subjective experience, with no right way or wrong to experience it or respond to it" (p. 18). Since music therapists have spent most of their lives actively involved in making music, studying music, and performing music, they understand first hand how important music can be in one's life. Client responses will be varied, both in individual and group settings. Music therapists must acknowledge in a nonjudgmental manner the perceived positive and negative experiences of clients to therapist-selected music.

Client-Selected Music

While the music therapist often selects music for listening experiences, the client or group can select the music to be heard. A client's music is familiar and has an established relationship. In comparison with therapist-selected music, a client-selected song provides a higher degree of predictability and control for the client. They likely know the music and believe they understand how they will react to hearing the song. For some clients, adolescent clients in particular, the opportunity to "control" the situation by selecting the music can improve rapport between client and music therapist.

Song selection may reveal subconscious feelings for the person who cannot verbally express feelings (Vaughn, 1993). Vaughn (1993) reported,

> Data pertaining to the psychology of the mind, the neuroanatomy of the human brain, and the clinical experiences of scores of music therapists lend support to a theory that songs provide an outlet for the expression of conscious and subconscious feelings. (p. 23)

The selection of songs may inform the music therapist of the client's progress in therapy. The level of insight a client possesses is often evident in the selections brought to music therapy. For example, a person in treatment for drug abuse who brings in a song glorifying the abuse of chemicals is not likely focused on the goals of his or her treatment. However, if the person brings a song about loss or regret over failed relationships, he or she is possibly developing insight into the consequences of his or her actions.

Other Uses of Music—Structured Recreation

Music therapists often work in privately or state-funded psychiatric facilities that provide both acute and long-term treatment and inpatient and day treatments. These programs often limit a client's access to music. People needing psychiatric care may choose inappropriate ways to use music or ways that exacerbate their illness. Due to the symptoms of the client's illness or side effects of medications, he or she may lack the attention span needed to enjoy music. Just as music therapists select experiences with music to engage clients in the therapy process, they can also structure music experience for recreation, fun, and leisure skill development. Techniques include ensemble participation, such as a chorus, hand bell choirs, or rock band, and learning to play an instrument for leisure. Active participation, a sense of belonging, and attention to task are important skills in recovering from mental illness. Music is an attractive venue for practicing these skills. Structured music for recreation can provide stimulation and sensory involvement for a highly sterile environment or provide order in a chaotic environment.

A Word of Caution

A word of caution is appropriate at this point. If people are restricted from listening to any music in a program, music can become even more powerful. Tom, a client in a substance abuse program, once stated to the author, "I'll do anything you want in group to have music!" Another client, a young woman named Louise with an acute psychotic depression, expressed the impact of music on a readmission screening. The woman had attended two or three group music therapy sessions in an acute treatment unit. Louise sat near the edge of the group and only commented if directly questioned. Her affect rarely changed from its fixed state. She was discharged after five days in the hospital. She returned shortly after her discharge seeking readmission.

The admission counselor reported that Louise said she wanted to "go back where the music was." Music and music experiences are powerful and wonderful tools for connecting with clients, but should not be used without careful consideration and understanding. A psychotherapist would carefully consider the use of hypnosis or free association with a patient. Yet, because music is so common and seemingly benign, it can be easily misused or underused.

Songs in Music Therapy

A specific type of music used in music therapy is the song. A song generally refers to a work that has lyrics, a melodic line, and an accompanying harmonic structure. Documented successes of using song in music therapy include treating women with eating disorders (Hilliard, 2001a; Parente, 1989), survivors of sexual abuse (Clendenon-Wallen, 1991; Lindberg, 1995; Mayers, 1995), adult psychiatry (Ficken, 1976), adults with chemical dependency (Freed, 1987), adults who are HIV positive and depressed (Cordobes, 1997), and adults in grief counseling (Wexler, 1989). Songs and music play an integral role in the lives and identity development of adolescents (Clendenon-Wallen, 1991; James, 1990; Kennelly, 2001) and frequently represent the values of a generation (White, 1985). Songs in therapy have been used in the treatment of adolescents with substance abuse issues (James, 1990) and adolescents with emotional disturbance (Edgerton, 1990).

Singing Songs

One use of composed songs in therapy is the sing-along in which clients sing familiar and favorite songs. Singing familiar and identified favorite songs supports the development of the therapeutic rapport between therapist and client (Goldstein, 1990; Kennelly, 2001). Familiar songs have established connections for the person and may remind the client of a healthier self, before the need for treatment (Edwards, 1998). Familiar songs generally elicit positive emotional reactions (Bryant, 1987). Singing songs can stimulate both the body and the emotions. The experience of singing can be viewed as fun and pleasurable, even when used in a therapy setting associated with pain and stress (Edwards, 1998; Hilliard, 2001a). The physical act of singing requires focused breathing and engages the muscles in the face.

These physical sensations may be understimulated in a person with a depressed mood and affect.

Analysis of Songs with Lyrics

Another technique using songs in therapy involves the analysis and discussion of song lyrics. Song lyrics are a medium that presents life's difficulties in a direct but nonthreatening manner (Mark, 1988; Schiff & Frances, 1974). The song's lyrics are fused with the stimulation provided by the music. Galizio and Hendrick (1972) found in a study that statements reflecting issues of the time were better received when sung or accompanied by guitar music. The music may have created positive emotional arousal leaving the subjects more receptive to the information.

Analysis of popular song lyrics can influence perceived locus of control in adolescents in recovery from substance abuse (James, 1990), assist in identifying cognitive distortions in women with eating disorders (Hilliard, 2001a), and may be used as a lead-in intervention prior to writing songs with clients (Ficken, 1976; Freed, 1987; Edgerton, 1990). Song lyrics are useful within cognitive therapy frameworks as music lyrics can be used to identify cognitive distortions (Selm, 1991). Within the Gestalt framework, song and song lyrics can serve as transitional objects (Diaz de Chumaceiro, 1992). Wexler (1989) reported, "Songs may have functioned as a familiar medium with which the clients were able to identify" (p. 65). According to a publication by Vaughn (1993), this ability to relate to song lyrics may be useful for persons who "are unable or unwilling to communicate their feelings verbally and consciously" (p. 22). Discussion of song lyrics provides a safe, confrontative tool.

Songs in storytelling format allow clients in therapy to "empathize with the principal character's feelings and in doing so project their own feelings" (Clendenon-Wallen, 1991, p. 78). The therapist may either select songs that identify issues of treatment or have the client identify the songs. The client's ability to recognize issues and express them through music may be evident in the song selection. If a suitable song cannot be located, music therapists can write a song with pertinent lyrics in order to meet the needs of individual clients (Robb, 1996; Wexler, 1989).

Songwriting

Music therapists assist clients in writing songs in therapy, and song-writing is well documented as a therapeutic technique (Edgerton, 1990; Ficken, 1976; Freed, 1987; Goldstein, 1990; Schmidt, 1983). Song-writing creates a product, a finished song, but the process of the song-writing is the focus of music therapy (Clendenon-Wallen, 1991; Cordobes, 1997; Edgerton, 1990; Ficken, 1976; Freed, 1987; Lindberg, 1995; Schmidt, 1983). The process of writing songs or creating music and lyr-ics through improvisation is selected to achieve a number of clinical goals, including increased verbal communication, increased socializa-tion and interaction among group members (Hilliard, 2001a; Robb, 1996), improved self-concept and self-esteem (Edgerton, 1990; Freed, 1987; Lindberg, 1995), increasing self-expression and the expression of feelings (Clendenon-Wallen, 1991; Cordobes, 1997; Goldstein, 1990; Kennelly, 2001), and an increased sense of cohesion among group mem-bers (Cordobes, 1997; Freed, 1987). Songwriting techniques can be in-corporated into a cognitive therapy framework to identify cognitive distortions, and processing modes, and to identify irrational beliefs (Bryant, 1987; Hilliard, 2001a; Luce, 2001; Selm, 1991). The construc-tion of a song communicates with the metaphorical and synthesizing parts of the brain—a process important in achieving change (Selm, 1991).

Though songs written in therapy often focus on a client's struggles and negative emotions, the result of the process may elicit feelings of pride and accomplishment when the newly created song is complete. The song product may allow clients to leave their negative experi-ences in the song (Edwards, 1998). Songwriting reduced feelings of frustration and guilt in clients recovering from substance abuse (Jones, 1998). Writing one's own lyrics to songs helps clients resolve conflicts that have been challenging in his or her life. This chance for resolution is a benefit of songwriting techniques.

The musical responsibilities in songwriting fall upon the music therapist. In a technique referred to as song augmentation or "piggy-backing" (Edwards, 1998; Ficken, 1976; Schmidt, 1983), a familiar tune serves as the musical structure for which new lyrics are written. A group can compose original lyrics using a number of techniques, including word association techniques (Lindberg, 1995), theme selection following lyric analysis of existing songs (Edgerton, 1990), and general "brainstorming." Once song lyrics have been completed, the music therapist may play different styles of musical accompaniment and allow the group to choose one that fits the song (Cordobes, 1997; Lindberg, 1995; Schmidt, 1983). Though most of the song-writing research reports on songs written within a single session, song components may be separated and spread over several sessions (Edgerton, 1990). Song writing in music therapy provides a flexible technique for self-expression and problem solving while providing the immediate reward of a finished song.

Music-Assisted Relaxation

Another common use of music within the psychotherapy framework is music-assisted relaxation. Training clients in relaxation methods can be useful for their recovery. Music therapists often provide music-assisted relaxation training for reducing stress and providing anxiety management (Wolfe, 2000). Unkefer (1990) wrote that the music stimulus diverts the client's attention away from unpleasant sensations, such as tension, anxiety, and agitation, while allowing "a safe and pleasant perceptual experience" through focus on the music (p. 169). While music therapists can provide live music for relaxation, the majority of music-assisted relaxation practices by music therapists includes selected, recorded music. The benefits of using recorded music include the opportunity for the participant to purchase the same recording and practice the techniques outside of the therapy setting. Music therapy interventions for stress and anxiety management include music listening, music listening combined with physically based relaxation techniques (Robb, 2000), music and deep breathing (Strauser, 1997), and music and imagery for relaxation (Sedei Godley, 1987). The music therapist's training in music allows him or her to understand the rhythmic and harmonic organization of the music and tailor the relaxation method to the music and for the individual client.

The selection of music for relaxation purposes requires the same care and attention as selecting music for emotional recovery needs. A person's musical preference and past experiences, particularly musical training, will significantly influence the ability of the music to promote relaxation. Standley's 1996 meta-analysis found that music that is slow and nonvocal generally lowers the physiological symptoms of stress, though significant intersubjective differences were noted. Davis and Thaut (1989) studied the effects of subject-selected music on perceived anxiety and level of relaxation. Subjects in the study listened to music from their own collections that included rock and roll, folk music, and contemporary Christian music, all genres containing music that would not be considered slow and nonvocal. They reported feeling relaxed after listening to their preferred music with a significant reduction in self-reported anxiety. Physiological measures, however, showed that this music aroused the autonomic nervous system (Davis & Thaut, 1989). Hanser (1985) conducted an extensive literature review on music for relaxation. She found that there was a correlation between liking the music and reported relaxation. Client preferences appear to play a significant role in music listening for relaxation.

Music therapists look for certain characteristics in music that promote a state of relaxation. Music for relaxation should be as calming as possible. There should be few surprises in the music. Drastic changes from soft to loud music, such as from violins to trumpets, should be avoided. The brain is alerted to changes and "lulled to sleep" by monotony (Jourdain, 1997). The fact that a person's preferred music has a relaxing quality, even if the characteristics are alerting, may be due to its familiarity. Music that is familiar to a listener due to repeated hearings or seems predictable by its consistent elements of rhythm and harmony may provide this needed monotony. Music is ordered in time and has a foreseeable (fore-hear-able) end. Allowing oneself to relax may cause an altered sense of time. Music orders time and alerts the listener to the end. This predictability can be comforting.

Conversely, the music must not fail to capture and maintain the attention of the listener. Boredom leads to distraction, which interferes with relaxation. If the client-therapist relationship is strong, the presence of the music therapist may provide an element of familiarity and predictability. Trust in the relaxation process may be an extension of trust in the therapist and may facilitate relaxation.

Thaut and Davis (1993) found that over 80 percent of the subjects relaxing by listening to music incorporated other strategies to assist with relaxation, such as deep breathing, muscle relaxation, and imagery. While the college students who served in the study incorporated these techniques without instruction, music therapists may need to coach clients in using these techniques with music. Robb (2000) compared music-assisted progressive muscle relaxation, traditional progressive muscle relaxation without music, music listening, and a period of silence for effectiveness in reducing anxiety and promoting relaxation. She found no significant differences among the techniques, but the music-assisted progressive muscle relaxation had the greatest change in scores from pretest to posttest. Other interesting factors discovered in the study include the fact that subjects reported more random thoughts and fatigue responses during music listening and silence periods. The music-assisted progressive muscle relaxation provided the greatest relaxation response with less reported sleepiness after the relaxation exercise. Standley et al. (2004) reported that the benefits of progressive relaxation techniques increased with the addition of music.

Music's use of tension and release can be paired with deep breathing exercises for relaxation. Deep breathing can be timed with music. Imagery related to the breath, such as inhaling warmth or light, can be paired with music that supports the imagery. Other imagery scripts can be generated by the music therapist and used for relaxation. Scripts often include imagining favorite places, such as the beach or the mountains, engaging in favorite activities, or relaxing sensations, such as floating or rocking. Music is selected to promote an imagery experience that brings about relaxation.

The use of music in relaxation training pairs music and pleasure. While music's inherently pleasurable qualities interfere with the consideration of music as an unconditioned stimulus, the pairing of specific music and relaxation training may condition the music to evoke a relaxation response in the absence of the music therapist and therapy session. Therefore, if the music becomes a conditioned stimulus, the patient can play the music at times of stress and receive the benefits of relaxation. Music-assisted relaxation techniques can be used within a cognitive/behavioral therapy framework, as well as other psychotherapy approaches (Darrow, 2004).

Creating Music Through Improvisation

Creating music in therapy provides an in-the-moment experience of creation and expression. It also provides greater freedom and more unknowns. It creates a musical product—a song or improvised music.

In scenario #1, drumming is an example of improvised, or spontaneous, music. The music therapist structured the initial experience to make it accessible, but allowed each person the freedom to play as he or she chose during the eight silent beats. The client was invited to play anything on the drum—loudly or softly, fast or slow, aggressively or timidly, or play nothing at all. Such a task can be challenging for a client with low self-esteem, or who is in a manic state, or who controls every aspect of life. The musical process allows for ineffective and coping behaviors to present themselves in the therapy session. The music experience acts like a mirror, often revealing the causes that led a person to therapy.

Music improvisation in therapy offers a wealth of experiences and intervention levels. Improvised music is often associated with jazz music, but is something most of us have done and can do. Children create spontaneous melodies and songs as they play. Adults often hurry children out the door with a chant, repeating the words "let's go" several times in a rhythmic manner. We often find ourselves tapping out rhythms with pencils as we daydream at the computer screen and repeating rhythms that we find entertaining. People create music spontaneously, but creating music on "demand" in a therapy session is less common. The music therapist is trained in structuring the musical experience for the needs of the client.

Improvisation can be a solo from a client only or therapist only, a duet between client and therapist, or an ensemble in group therapy. The musical demand upon a client can range from volunteering a single note or word to playing a 30-minute solo improvisation. Music can be improvisation on any instrument, with the voice, or even the body, such as clapping hands, stomping feet, or snapping fingers. Music therapists may ask clients to improvise music that represents an emotion, situation, or other "nonmusical" topic. Such music is referred to as a referential improvisation (Bruscia, 2001), other times, creating meaningful, organized music without any referential topic may be the focus. Improvisation creates a product, which may be recorded and played back for analysis by the client and/or the therapist. Musical compositions can be given titles, verbal descriptions, or used to stimulate verbal processing. Bruscia's 1987 book titled, *Improvisational Models of Music Therapy,* is the most thorough work on improvised music therapy.

Music improvisation addresses a number of therapeutic goals. Self-expression and self-exploration are commonly identified with the technique. A participant's ability to organize is evident in music improvisation. In group improvisation, interaction among the players and with the therapist will illuminate problems and coping strategies. Improvisation can be a completely nonverbal technique and structured to avoid verbalization and possible intellectualization (Nolan, 1989).

The case study of "Nadine," a 16-year-old girl, may provide some insight into the benefits of music improvisation in therapy. Following a suicide attempt, Nadine was admitted to the adolescent unit of a psychiatric hospital. She was diagnosed with ongoing depression. Her parents were divorced and each had remarried. She lived in one parent's home for a week and spent the following week in the home of the other parent. She literally had two houses, two bedrooms, and two different sets of parents and siblings. Nadine attended group music therapy sessions two times a week where she was cooperative, though guarded. In lyric analysis, she chose the literal description of emotion in song lyrics (when I'm sad I cry) and drew cartoon-like symbols of teardrops on her papers. She maintained restricted affect, seemed to disappear in groups, and offered little verbal dialogue.

In order to provide outlets for emotional expression, she was referred for one-to-one music therapy. Music improvisation was chosen as a primary intervention since it offered her nonverbal expression. She was asked by the music therapist to play music about her feelings, her life, and her recent suicide attempt. She chose as instruments for herself, a soprano xylophone (higher tones) and some small shakers. The music therapist chose a bass range xylophone (lower tones) for support. Until the therapist played a strong, repeated bass pattern, Nadine's music was timid, soft, and limited in organization as evidenced by her randomly picking out notes or switching instruments. The therapist's supportive, musical grounding seemed to provide her with what she was lacking. Her melodies and rhythms began to flow more easily, and she could sustain a single idea for several minutes. As she played, her energy level and posture improved.

Despite continuing to need the support of the therapist's musical grounding for successful improvisation, she was discharged after completing two more music therapies. A second suicide attempt followed a few days later and she was readmitted to the psychiatric facility. She resumed both group and individual music therapy. Her second admission prompted strong family therapy interventions. Her final session's music signified her emotional changes. As she chose instruments for improvisation, she selected the bass xylophone typically used by the therapist. She gave the therapist her soprano xylophone. Nadine organized the music with her bass line and provided the foundation for the improvisation. Limited verbal processing was necessary. She was now able to ground herself. She did not return to the hospital.

The Bonny Method of Guided Imagery and Music

Music therapy is a highly flexible approach. Music improvisation offers numerous experiences with different instruments and use of the voice, using both referential methods and musical methods and in group or individual settings. The Bonny method of GIM may appear to be the most "scripted" process in music therapy. Music is chosen by the therapist and is exclusively classical music from the Western art music tradition. Sessions have four basic phases, a preliminary conversation where the process is explained (first session only) and goals are set, an induction where a state of relaxation is facilitated, a music program where a selected music is played while the client travels to the music and reports his or her imagery, and a post session integration or review in which the client returns to an alert state and images are processed (Burns & Woolrich, 2004). GIM is a powerful process and only recommended for clients who are capable of symbolic thinking and can differentiate between symbolic thinking and reality (Bonny, 1994). It is not recommended for people experiencing any form of psychosis.

Guided imagery and music evolved in the 1970s when psychedelic drugs were being used clinically. Psychedelic drugs were reportedly capable of enhancing self-awareness and bringing about a catharsis (Bonny, 1994). According to him,

> Meanwhile, explorations in the use of relaxation and a prepared tape of music selections had begun to bring surprising results. Therapeutically meaningful imagery was evoked by careful application of classical music, and this approach was sometime more effective than the longer, more intense drug sessions. (p. 70)

The first book concerning GIM, *Music and Your Mind,* was written by Helen Bonny and Louis Savary. The technique of GIM is similar to psychoanalysis during which the client lies on a couch or the floor and reports images to the therapist. During GIM, classical music is used as the stimulus to generate images because it is "able to provide the depth of experience, variety of color and form, harmonic and melodic complexity which are qualities needed for self-exploration" (Bonny, 1994, p. 73). This description of classical music using words like complexity and variety, strikingly contrasts the slow, nonvocal, and calming description of music for relaxation.

The bachelor's degree in music therapy does not include training in GIM. In order to become a fellow, a practitioner of GIM endorsed by the Association for Music and Imagery (AMI), a training process of approximately three years is necessary. GIM training encompasses both didactic and in-depth experiential work in psychotherapy. Bonny (1994) describes the ideal candidate for training in GIM as "mature life-experienced." Though a number of GIM practitioners are also board certified as music therapists, being a music therapist is not a requirement. Fellows include those who have studied clinical psychology and creative arts therapies. GIM training was first established in 1975 and is now offered in the United States, England, New Zealand, Australia, and several other countries. Populations treated with GIM include individuals with AIDS, people with borderline personalities, people with depression, and people seeking self-awareness (Peters, 2000). GIM is a specific procedure using classical music to create an imagery experience that is reported to a guide in a didactic therapy format.

CONCLUSION

Music therapy techniques encompass actively listening to music, the use of songs, analysis of song lyrics, writing original songs, improvised music, music-assisted relaxation, and GIM. Music therapy can fit into a number of psychotherapeutic approaches. Music therapists tailor music experiences to the specific needs of clients and are mindful of the personal nature of music experiences. Music's strong appeal and its links to pleasurable experiences make it useful in a behavioral approach. Music in therapy techniques, such as lyric analysis or song writing, using verbal processing can be adapted to cognitive, analytical, or reality therapy methods. Music therapists work effectively as a part of interdisciplinary teams. Music therapy may be the emotional outlet needed by a client to express feelings, confront cognitive distortions, provide the relaxation that enables effective work in individual therapy, or identify a leisure outlet for using free time constructively.

LEVELS OF TREATMENT

Techniques used in music therapy are adapted to meet the needs of the level of treatment, whether the treatment modality is inpatient or outpatient, voluntary or involuntary, crisis intervention or ongoing therapy. Several levels of music therapy practice exist. The level of treatment is influenced by two primary factors—the intensity of the relationship between client and therapist and the client's emotional and cognitive abilities. As the person's acute symptoms subside and the client-therapist relationship strengthens, more intense levels of therapy may become appropriate. The desired outcome of the therapy is also considered. The needs for crisis intervention and in-depth, ongoing therapy are different and require different levels of therapeutic intensity.

The first level of treatment is labeled supportive music psychotherapy by Bruscia (1998) and called music therapy as activity therapy by Wheeler (1983). The focus of this level of music therapy is to reduce symptoms, strengthen coping skills, and remain in the moment. It involves using structured music experiences to influence behavioral changes, rather than seeking an understanding of why behaviors exist in the person (Peters, 2000). It is effective as a crisis intervention, as an early intervention, or for people whose symptoms prevent deeper work, such as individuals suffering with psychosis, severe depression, or medication side effects.

An example of a technique adaptable to the supportive or activity therapy level is the sing-along. An individual selects songs from a songbook or song list to sing either as an individual or in a group situation. The music therapist sings the songs with the client(s) and accompanies the singing with guitar or piano. While the songs selected by each member have significance, the goals at this level of treatment are on choosing, listening or singing, and attending to the music. The music therapist supports the clients in making choices of songs that are helpful in maintaining a "here and now" focus on the music. For example, if the tone of a selection appears to be counterproductive to the goals of the group, the therapist may ask the client or group to choose another song to sing. Limited verbal discussion of why each song was chosen is offered or encouraged.

The next level of treatment is called insight music psychotherapy by Bruscia (1998), insight music therapy with reeducative goals by Wheeler (1983), and process-oriented music therapy by Davis, Gfeller, and Thaut (1999). During this level of treatment, music experiences are used to identify and express feelings, explore coping skills, experience problem solving, and verbally process such experiences. Insight/process oriented music therapy requires that participants be oriented to reality and be able to communicate with others. Feelings and self-awareness are dealt with on a conscious level with a focus on the here and now experience with the music (Wheeler, 1983). Verbal processing plays an important role in the treatment. The sing-along intervention can be easily adapted and used in an insight-oriented experience. The therapist may ask each person to choose a song about how they feel at that moment or one that conveys an emotion they need to explore. The music therapist sings and accompanies the group. Verbal discussion about the music experience may include the emotions experienced during the song or in reaction to the song, why the song was chosen, and the feedback shared among group members. Dialogue focuses on present emotions and experiences in the conscious memory as a result of the music experience. Feedback among group members may be encouraged.

A more intense level of music therapy is called insight-oriented music therapy with reconstructive goals by Wheeler (1983) and reconstructive, analytically and catharsis-oriented music therapy by Davis, Gfeller, and Thaut (1999). This level of music therapy uses music and music experiences to recover unconscious material and reconstruct the personality. Since the majority of music therapists practice with a bachelor's degree, advanced training is recommended for this level of treatment and clinical supervision at this level of treatment is appropriate. While the sing-along technique could be adapted for this level of practice, it is limited in its ability to elicit images from the unconscious. A client could select songs that reflect a particular childhood conflict, but more often improvisation or music and imagery experiences would be selected. The participant must be reality oriented, the client-therapist relationship must be strong, and the participant must be motivated to maximize this level of therapy.

MUSIC IN *THERAPY OR MUSIC* AS *THERAPY*

Music can be used *in* therapy, in conjunction with verbal and other techniques, or *as* therapy, where the primary therapeutic mode is the music experience. One type of music *as* therapy is called by Bruscia (1998) transformative music psychotherapy. He wrote

> the therapist uses music experiences and the relationships that form through them in order to access, work through, and resolve the client's therapeutic needs; verbal techniques are used only if or when they will enhance the music experience and the therapeutic potential . . . the music experience is therapeutically transformative and complete in, of, and by itself. . . . (p. 219)

Bruscia references techniques such as the Bonny method of GIM as those used in transformative music psychotherapy. Music-assisted relaxation and structured music recreation are also examples of music as therapy. Music as therapy relies on the music to bring about changes with limited verbal process. Music *in* therapy, in contrast, uses music experiences to facilitate the verbal process. Music therapists work with both frameworks.

CASE STUDIES

Donnie—Music Therapy and Reflection of Self-Organization

Donnie was an eight-year-old boy admitted to the children's unit of a psychiatric hospital after cutting his foster mother with a knife. He had been abused by a number of adults. He was the victim of sexual abuse from his biological mother and of neglect and torture from a previous set of foster parents. He and his siblings had been removed from their biological parents and sent to separate foster systems. The hospital unit used a strongly behavioral approach to treatment using a level system. Donnie was frequently in "time-out" due to his inability to control his emotions and aggressive behavior. He attended small group music therapy (four to five children) in which he was not successful. Attempts to manage his aggression and impulsivity with medications failed. Trials on antipsychotic medication caused severe rashes as side effects. As all medications wore off, an obsessive-compulsive tendency became evident. Donnie would attack roommates who failed to keep the room orderly. When it became necessary to separate Donnie from his peers, individual music therapy was recommended.

As a part of the music therapy assessment, instruments were placed on the floor ready for use in music improvisation. Donnie entered the room and immediately lined the instruments up end-to-end across the floor. He then played each one down the line in order. He seemed completely unaware that the therapist was playing music with him. The music therapist and Donnie sat at the piano in order to improvise music. He played loudly on a cluster of keys with little variation, again seemingly unaware of the therapist. When asked how the music would stop, he yelled, "Stop!" and removed his hands. His musical expressions had no organization—no discernible melody, harmony, or rhythm. The only organizational system he had was externalized and involved lining up the instruments. A final improvisation was shared between Donnie and the music therapist. Two xylophones with removable keys were placed on the floor facing each other. Donnie spent considerable time removing and replacing the keys on both instruments, without testing the different sounds of the instrument with different key combinations. Once he was satisfied with the visual organization, he began to strike the remaining keys. The music therapist joined him. Once again he seemed oblivious to the therapist's attempts to interact musically. The therapist hit his instrument with a mallet, violating his "space" in a large gesture. He made eye contact for the first time and laughed. This "violation" became a game that ended the sessions.

Donnie's musical behaviors were a clear reflection of how he organized his life. As a reflection of his sustained abuse by adults, he only noticed the therapist after his musical space was violated. His disorganized display of sounds indicated his lack of internal organization. He organized his music physically, by arranging the instruments or bars on the xylophone, much like he organized his room in his compulsive way. His "misbehaviors" on the children's unit, aggression and intrusion into other's space, could better be defined in terms of his need for external order. If other children exerted their will and disturbed his sense of order, he retaliated. He continued in the final three sessions to make connection with the music therapist in improvisation only if his instrument was struck or some physical boundary was challenged. Donnie was transferred to a long-term program to continue therapy.

Stacie—Music As a Behavioral Reward Within a Self-Exploration Framework

Stacie was a high school drop out who had just turned 18. She was diagnosed as having a borderline personality disorder with recurrent major depression. She had been admitted a number of times to the psychiatric center following suicide attempts and episodes of running away and engaging in risky behaviors. Due to her immaturity and seductive behavior around older males, she was placed on the adolescent program. She was hospitalized during a holiday season and for a few days was the only patient in the adolescent program. Stacie tended to exhaust staff members with clinginess and her maudlin nature. Despite most staff members' attempts to meet her with positive regard, she was challenging. It was discovered that she wrote song lyrics; the staff brought this to the music therapist's attention. Stacie not only wrote lyrics, but, despite her lack of formal music training, also had constructed original melodies for her songs. Her lyrics were insightful, expressing her emotional struggles with lines such as "cast away like nobody cares" and "I'm longing to belong somewhere." She articulated her difficult transition into adulthood, her perceived lack of support from her adoptive mother, and her struggles with depression.

The treatment team decided upon an approach rewarding Stacie's coping skills and positive behavior, rather than dwelling on her ongoing personality diffusion and attention-seeking behaviors that dramatized negative emotions. The songs provided an outlet through which to express negative emotions, but in a manner that made them manageable and separate from her self-identity. She received positive attention and sincere praise for her songwriting ability. She enjoyed adding guitar accompaniment to her songs and recording them with the music therapist. Whenever negative behaviors or attempts at manipulation surfaced, Stacie was reminded that she would lose her chance to record her songs. As more sincere interactions were possible, the attitude of the staff changed toward Stacie. Stacie was less one-dimensional, and became more than just a rejected, sad, clingy person. The staff related to her through her songs and the process of song writing, rather than through the exhausting verbal dialogue focused on her "suffering." The process of song writing and recording was both a reward and a therapy. Not only did Stacie's songs change the staff members' view of her, but also she began to accept a more positive view of herself.

SUMMARY STATEMENT

Music therapy capitalizes on the social nature of the music experience, the elements of music to structure experience and brain activity, and the use of music to create and experience a therapeutic relationship. Music therapy is an individualized treatment provided by a board certified music therapist. The music serves as a functional tool working toward behavior changes in clients that promote wellness. Music therapists assess the needs of the client within a bio-psycho-social framework, establish the goals and objectives for treatment, design music experiences for the client within the therapeutic relationship, document outcomes, and evaluate treatment. Models of music therapy as psychotherapy range from psychoanalytic to cognitive/behavior and are effective in short-term and long-term therapy protocols. Music therapists work collaboratively with other therapists and in multidisciplinary treatment. Perhaps the following statement by Maureen Draper (2001) can summarize the unique therapeutic contribution of music. She wrote,

At times music brings the gift of self-forgetting, inviting us to slip out of our own skin. But paradoxically, because it connects with our emotions, music often brings more self-awareness. And it's easier to meet our own emotions when we meet them in music. (p. 9)

REFERENCES

Alvin, J.A. (1975). *Music therapy.* New York: Basic Books, Inc.

American Music Therapy Association (1999). Frequently asked questions about music therapy. Retrieved on June 30, 2003, from www.musictherapy.org/faqs .html#WHAT_DO_MUSIC_THERAPISTS_DO.

American Music Therapy Association (2001 November). Standards for Education and Clinical Training. Unpublished document presented at annual meeting of the AMTA in St. Louis, MO.

American Music Therapy Association (2003). *AMTA member sourcebook.* Silver Spring, MD: AMTA, Inc.

Blake, R.L. & Bishop, S.R. (1994). Bonny method of guided imagery and music (GIM) in the treatment of post-traumatic stress disorder (PTSD) in adults in the psychiatric setting. *Music Therapy Perspectives, 12*(2), 125-129.

Bonny, H.L. (1994). Twenty-one years later: A GIM update. *Music Therapy Perspectives, 12*(2), 70-74.

Boxill, E.H. (1985). *Music therapy for the developmentally disabled.* Rockville, MD: Aspen Systems.

Bruscia, K.E. (1987). *Improvisational models of music therapy.* Springfield, IL: Charles C. Thomas, Publisher.

Bruscia, K.E. (1998). *Defining music therapy* (2nd ed.). Gilsum, NH: Barcelona Publishers.

Bruscia, K.E. (2001). A qualitative approach to analyzing client improvisations. *Music Therapy Perspectives, 19,* 7-21.

Bryant, D. (1987). A cognitive approach to therapy through music. *Journal of Music Therapy, 34,* 27-34.

Burns, D. & Woolrich, J. (2004). The Bonny method of guided imagery in music. In A.A. Darrow (Ed.), *Introduction to approaches in music therapy* (pp. 53-62). Silver Spring, MD: American Music Therapy Association, Inc.

Butler, B. (1966). Music group psychotherapy. *Journal of Music Therapy, 3,* 53-56.

Certification Board for Music Therapists. (2003). Retrieved August 7, 2003, from www.cbmt.org.

Clendenon-Wallen, J. (1991). The use of music to influence the self-confidence and self-esteem of adolescents who are sexually abused. *Music Therapy Perspectives, 9,* 73-79.

Cordobes, T.K. (1997). Group songwriting as a method for developing group cohesion for HIV seropositive adult patients with depression. *Journal of Music Therapy, 34,* 46-67.

Darrow, A.A. (2004). *Introduction to approaches in music therapy.* Silver Spring, MD: American Music Therapy Association, Inc.

Davis, W.B. (1989). Music therapy in Victorian England: Frederick Kill Harford and the Guild of St. Cecilia. *Music Therapy Perspectives, 7,* 17-22.

Davis, W.B. (1996). An instruction course in the use and practice of music therapy: The first handbook of music therapy clinical practice. *Journal of Music Therapy, 33,* 34-46.

Davis, W.B., Gfeller, K.E., & Thaut, M.H. (1999). *An introduction to music therapy: Theory and practice* (2nd ed.). New York: McGraw-Hill College.

Davis, W.B. & Thaut, M.H. (1989). The influence of preferred relaxing music on measures of state anxiety, relaxation, and physiological responses. *Journal of Music Therapy, 24,* 168-187.

Diaz de Chumaceiro, C.L. (1992). Transference-countertransference in psychology integrations for music therapy in 1970s and 1980s. *Journal of Music Therapy, 29,* 217-235.

Dougherty, K.M. (1984). Music therapy in the treatment of the alcoholic client. *Music Therapy: The Journal of the American Association for Music Therapy, 4*(1), 47-54.

Draper, M.M. (2001). *The nature of music: Beauty, sound, and healing.* New York: Riverhead Books.

Dvorkin, J. (1982). Piano improvisation: A therapeutic tool in acceptance and resolution of emotions in a schizo-affective personality. *Music Therapy, 2*(1), 53-62.

Edgerton, C.D. (1990). Creative group songwriting. *Music Therapy Perspectives, 8,* 15-19.

Edwards, J. (1998). Music therapy for children with severe burns. *Music Therapy Perspectives, 16*(1), 21-26.

Farnsworth, P.R. (1969). *The social psychology of music* (2nd ed.). Ames, IA: Iowa State University Press.

Ficken, T. (1976). The use of songwriting in a psychiatric setting. *Journal of Music Therapy, 13,* 163-172.

Freed, B.S. (1987). Songwriting with the chemically dependent. *Music Therapy Perspectives, 4,* 13-18.

Friedlander, L.H. (1994). Group music psychotherapy in an inpatient psychiatric setting for children: A developmental approach. *Music Therapy Perspectives, 12*(2), 92-97.

Galizio, M. & Hendrick, C. (1972). Effect of musical accompaniment on attitude: The guitar as a prop for persuasion. *Journal of Applied Social Psychology, 2,* 350-359.

Goldstein, S.L. (1990). A songwriting assessment for hopelessness in depressed adolescents: A review of literature and a pilot study. *Arts in Psychotherapy, 17,* 117-124.

Grout, D.J. & Palisca, C.V. (1988). *A history of western music.* New York: W.W. Norton & Company, Inc.

Halpern, S. & Savary, L. (1985). *Sound health.* New York: Harper & Row, Publishers, Inc.

Hanser, S.B. (1985). Music therapy and stress reduction research. *Journal of Music Therapy, 22,* 193-206.

Hanser, S.B. (1987). *Music therapist's handbook.* St. Louis, MO: Warren H. Green, Inc.

Hilliard, R.E. (2001a). The use of cognitive-behavioral therapy in the treatment of women with eating disorders. *Music Therapy Perspectives, 19*(2), 109-113.

Hilliard, R.E. (2001b). The effects of music therapy–based bereavement groups on mood and behavior of grieving children: A pilot study. *Journal of Music Therapy, 38,* 291-306.

James, M.R. (1990). Adolescent values clarification: A positive influence on perceived locus of control. *Journal of Alcohol & Drug Education, 35*(2), 75-80.

James, M.R. & Freed, B.S. (1989). A sequential model for developing group cohesion in music therapy. *Music Therapy Perspectives, 7,* 28-34.

Jones, J.D. (1998). A comparison of songwriting and lyric analysis techniques to evoke emotional change in a single session with chemically dependent clients. Unpublished master's thesis, Florida State University.

Jourdain, R. (1997). *Music, the brain, and ecstasy: How music captures our imagination.* New York: Avon Books, Inc.

Justice, R.W. (1994). Music therapy interventions for people with eating disorders in an inpatient setting. *Music Therapy Perspectives, 12*(2), 104-110.

Kennelly, J. (2001). Music therapy in the bone marrow transplant unit: Providing emotional support during adolescence. *Music Therapy Perspectives, 19*(2), 104-108.

Kivland, M.J. (1986). The use of music to increase self-esteem in a conducted disordered adolescent. *Journal of Music Therapy, 23,* 25-29.

Lindberg, K.A. (1995). Songs of healing: Songwriting with an abused adolescent. *Music Therapy, 13*(1), 93-108.

Luce, D. (2001). Cognitive therapy and music therapy. *Music Therapy Perspectives, 19*(2), 96-103.

MacKay, J. (2002). Music therapy and mental health. Retrieved July 30, 2003, from www.mtabc.com.

Mark, A. (1988). Metaphoric lyrics as a bridge to the adolescent world. *Adolescence, 23,* 313-323.

Mayers, K.S. (1995). Songwriting as a way to decrease anxiety and distress in traumatized children. *The Arts in Psychotherapy, 22,* 495-498.

Murphy, M. (1983). Music therapy: A self-help group experience for substance abuse patients. *Music Therapy, 3*(1), 52-62.

Nolan, P. (1989). Music as a transitional object in the treatment of bulimia. *Music Therapy Perspectives, 6,* 49-51.

Parente, A.B. (1989). Feeding the hungry soul: Music as a therapeutic modality in the treatment of anorexia nervosa. *Music Therapy Perspectives, 6,* 44-48.

Pavlicevic, M., Trevarthen, C., & Duncan, J. (1994). Improvisational music therapy and the rehabilitation of persons suffering from chronic schizophrenia. *Journal of Music Therapy, 31,* 86-104.

Peters, J.S. (2000). *Music therapy: An introduction* (2nd ed.). Springfield, IL: Charles C Thomas.

Plach, T. (1980). *The creative use of music in group therapy.* Springfield, IL: Charles C Thomas.

Radocy, R.E. & Boyle, J.D. (1979). *Psychological foundations of musical behavior.* Springfield, IL: Charles C Thomas.

Richards, E. & Davies, A. (2002). Introduction. In E. Richards & A. Davies (Eds.), *Music therapy and group work* (pp. 15-26). Philadelphia, PA: Jessica Kingsley Publisher.

Rio, R.E. & Tenney, K.S. (2002). Music therapy for juvenile offenders in residential treatment. *Music Therapy Perspectives, 20*(2), 89-97.

Robb, S.L. (1996). Techniques in song writing: Restoring emotional and physical well being in adolescents who have been traumatically injured. *Music Therapy Perspectives, 14*(1), 30-37.

Robb, S.L. (2000). Music assisted progressive muscle relaxation, progressive muscle relaxation, music listening, and silence: A comparison of relaxation techniques. *Journal of Music Therapy, 37*, 2-21.

Schiff, M. & Frances, A. (1974). Popular music: A training catalyst. *Journal of Music Therapy, 11*, 33-40.

Schmidt, J.A. (1983). Songwriting as a therapeutic procedure. *Music Therapy Perspectives, 1*(2), 4-7.

Sedei Godley, C. (1987). The use of music therapy in pain clinics. *Music Therapy Perspectives, 4*, 24-28.

Selm, Mark E. (1991). Chronic pain: Three issues in treatment and implications for music therapy. *Music Therapy Perspectives, 9*, 91-97.

Standley, J.M. (1996). Music research in medical/dental treatments: An update of a prior meta-analysis. In C.E. Furman (Ed.), *Effectiveness of music therapy procedures: Documentation of research and clinical practice* (2nd ed.). Washington, DC: National Association for Music Therapy, Inc.

Standley, J.M., Johnson, C.M., Robb, S.L., Brownell, M.D., & Kim, S.-H. (2004). Behavioral approach to music therapy. In A.A. Darrow (Ed.), *Introduction to approaches in music therapy* (pp. 103-124). Silver Spring, MD: American Music Therapy Association, Inc.

Strauser, J.M. (1997). The effects of music versus silence on measures of state anxiety, perceived relaxation, and physiological responses of patients receiving chiropractic interventions. *Journal of Music Therapy, 34*, 88-105.

Thaut, M.H. (1989). Music therapy, affect modulation, and therapeutic change: Toward an integrative model. *Music Therapy Perspectives, 7*, 55-62.

Thaut, M.H. & Davis, W.G. (1993). The influence of subject-selected versus experimenter-chosen music on affect, anxiety, and relaxation. *Journal of Music Therapy, 30*, 210-233.

Titon, J.T. & Slobin, M. (2002). The music-culture as a world of music. In J.T. Titon (Ed.), *Worlds of music: An introduction to the music of the world's peoples.* (pp. 1-34). Belmont, CA: Wadsworth Group.

Treder-Wolff, J. (1990). Affecting attitudes: Music therapy in addictions treatment. *Music Therapy Perspectives, 8*, 67-71.

Tyson, F. (1987). Analytically-oriented music therapy in a case of generalized anxiety disorder. *Music Therapy Perspectives, 4*, 51-55.

Unkefer, R.F. (Ed.). (1990). *Music therapy in the treatment of adults with mental disorders.* New York: Schrimer Books.

Vaughn, V.A. (1993). Musical expressions of subconscious feelings: A clinical perspective. *Music Therapy Perspectives, 11*(1), 16-23.

Ventre, M.E. (1994). Healing the wounds of childhood abuse: A Guided Imagery and Music case study. *Music Therapy Perspectives, 12*(2), 98-103.

Warja, M. (1994). Sounds of music through the spiraling path of individuation: A Jungian approach to music psychotherapy. *Music Therapy Perspectives, 12*(2), 75-83.

Wexler, M.M.D. (1989). The use of song in grief therapy with Cibecue White Mountain Apaches. *Music Therapy Perspectives, 7,* 63-66.

Wheeler, B.L. (1983). A psychotherapeutic classification of music therapy practices: A continuum of procedures. *Music Therapy Perspectives, 1,* 8-12.

White, A. (1985). Meaning and effects of listening to popular music: Implications for counseling. *Journal of Counseling and Development, 64,* 65-69.

Winn, W.T., Crowe, B.J., & Moreno, J.J. (1989). Shamanism and music therapy: Ancient healing techniques in modern practice. *Music Therapy Perspectives, 7,* 67-71.

Wolfe, D.E. (2000). Group music therapy in acute mental health care: Meeting the demands of effectiveness and efficacy. In C.E. Furman (Ed.), *Effectiveness of music therapy procedures: Documentation of research and clinical practice,* (3rd ed.). (pp. 265-296). Silver Spring, MD: American Music Therapy Association, Inc.

Chapter 9

Therapists and Animals: Demystifying Animal-Assisted Therapy

Aubrey H. Fine
Pamela F. Beiler

They never talk about themselves but listen while you talk about yourself, and keep up the appearance of being interested in the conversation.

Jerome K. Jerome, English humorist

Companionship, pleasure, affection, nonjudgmental acceptance, love, connection to the outside world, a reason to live—these are just a few of the countless benefits enjoyed by those who share their lives with beloved pets. The American Veterinary Medical Association reports that an estimated 61.6 million dogs and 68.9 million cats live in U.S. households, and that 36.1 percent of U.S. homes have dogs while 31.6 percent have cats (Gonzalez, 2002). Other popular family pets include birds, rabbits, turtles, fish, or one of the endless variety of other animal companions. No longer playing subordinate roles in American households, many companion animals are considered family members (Albert & Bulcroft, 1988), and according to Young (2003), 83 percent of adults refer to themselves as "mommy" or "daddy" to their pets. Some pet owners even value their pets as highly as a spouse or a parent (Gunter, 1999).

A growing body of literature referenced throughout this chapter emphasizes the importance of the human-animal bond and the benefits of incorporating animals into the treatment of medical and mental

Introduction to Alternative and Complementary Therapies
doi:10.1300/5987_09

health conditions. By understanding both the underlying principles that make animal-assisted therapy an effective treatment and the basics of devising an animal-assisted therapy program, clinicians may incorporate animals into treatment in a way that is enjoyable and beneficial to clients, rewarding for practitioners, and respectful to the animals involved in therapy.

PEOPLE AND THEIR PETS

Many theories have been proposed to explain why people adore being around animals. One widely accepted hypothesis stems from attachment theory and the need for humans to protect and to be protected (Sable, 1995). Defined by Bowlby (1969, 1980) and Ainsworth (1989), attachment behavior is any form of behavior that results in a person attaining or maintaining proximity to some other clearly identified individual who is perceived as better able to cope with the world. The biological function attributed to the attachment is that of protection. Barba (1995) suggested that the roles of humans in relationship with their pets often parallel roles of human-human relationships, especially that of child and parent. Just as young children rely on their parents, pets must depend on their human companions for continual care such as feeding and walking, or as protection from dangerous situations. Archer (1997) agreed with Barba's position and further noted that "people view relationships with pets similar to those of children" (p. 241). Many pet owners are often observed playing with their pets as parents would with their children and talking to them in "baby talk" or what Hirsch-Pasek and Treiman (1982) called "motherese."

A revealing survey examining respondents' attachment relationships with their pets found that 67 percent of respondents had a photograph of their dog, 73 percent let their pet sleep in the bedroom, and 40 percent celebrated the pet's birthday (Friedman, Katcher, Thomas, Lynch, & Messant, 1983). Even greater attachment to pets was found among single adults and others who are have fewer human ties compared to those with families (Albert & Bulcroft, 1988). Many cat owners ranked their cats higher than their husbands in unconditional love and affection (Zasloff & Kidd, 1994).

Pet owners commonly view their relationships with animals in humanistic terms. Many seem to develop anthropomorphic attitudes toward their pets, projecting onto the animals their own human feelings, motives, and qualities, and often perceiving pets as substitutes for other people (Selby & Rhoades, 1981). McNicholas and Collis (1995) pointed out advantages to the human/animal bond. They suggested that some people may become more attached to animals than to humans since they perceive their pets as always being available to meet their needs. The authors also noted that it often appears easier for humans to bond with animals than with other humans—unlike most humans, pets are typically indifferent to their human companions' material possessions, status, well-being, and social skills. It is possible that pets can provide an escape from the strains of human interaction.

ANIMALS AND HEALING

As noted by a growing body of research, animals can promote human physical and emotional wellness simply by being part of our lives. The demonstrated healing impact of animals on humans has been observed in both clinical and nonclinical settings with humans facing various physical and emotional challenges. A review of the numerous healing aspects of animals facilitates an understanding of how and why incorporating animals into therapeutic interventions can effectively lead to positive outcomes for a wide range of clients.

Physical Benefits

Animals can promote human physical wellness in a number of ways. A pioneer study led by Friedman, Katcher, Lynch, and Thomas (1980) concluded that among people with equally severe diseases, pet owners were less likely to die than those without pets. The seminal work of Gannt, the only American disciple of Pavlov and Lynch, led to the observation that blood pressure seems to rise when we speak with other humans and fall when we interact with animals (Lynch & McCarthy, 1969). More recently, Allen (2003) found that people with borderline hypertension had lower blood pressure on days when their dogs accompanied them to work.

Pet owners, especially dog owners, also appeared to have better physical health resulting from engaging in more cardio-activities and exercise than those without pets, and seniors with adopted pets reported a decrease in the frequency of minor health problems such as headaches, painful joints, hay fever, difficulty paying attention, colds and flu, dizziness, or kidney and bladder problems (Siegel, 1993). Montague (1995) also found that including animals and plants as an aspect of treatment in nursing home facilities led to a substantial reduction in medication costs, which dropped from an average of $3.80 per day to just $1.18 per day.

Psychosocial Benefits

Companion animals can also generate major psychosocial benefits. Pets tend to protect their human companions against stress, act as a social catalyst, and provide social support (McNicholas & Collis, 1995). Hunt, Hart, and Gomulkiewicz (1992) and Messant (1984) found that animals stimulate people to become more social and begin conversations with strangers. Steffens and Bergler (1988) reported that dog ownership fulfills numerous needs including social stimulation and an outlet for leisure. Muschel (1985) further explained that a pet could mitigate feelings of loneliness, loss, or displacement during transition periods such as moving to an unfamiliar area, losing a spouse, or a child leaving home.

Pets may play the roles of a friend, confidant, or even a family member. Bossard (1944) described animals as a source of unconditional love, an outlet for people's desire to express love, a teacher for children on topics such as toilet training, sex education, and as a companion. Pets can also facilitate communication either as nonjudgmental listeners through sounds or movements, or as catalysts for discussions among family members.

The presence of pets also appears to lead to decreased aggressive behaviors. A study conducted at Lima State Hospital by Lee (1984) found that on the wards with animals, there was a noticeable reduction in the patients' violent acts and attempted suicide, and the animals appeared to have a calming effect on the residents.

Several studies specifically point out psychosocial benefits that apply to seniors in the company of animals. Mugford and M'Comisky (1975) found significantly improved social attitudes and greater happiness among seniors who were given a parakeet for five months as compared to a control group. Pet ownership also appears to motivate seniors to perform activities of daily living such as getting out of bed and getting dressed due to a heightened sense of responsibility and of feeling needed by their pet (Raina et al., 1999). A study by Hart (1993) found that seniors who owned dogs took twice as many walks as nonowners, spoke more of their present lives rather than events of the past, and reported less dissatisfaction with their social, physical, and emotional state.

Among the numerous psychological benefits of human-animal interaction is a reduction in psychiatric symptoms such as decreased depression and anxiety (Garrity & Stallones, 1998). When required to perform a stressful task, women who participated in a study led by Allen, Blascovich, Tomaka, and Kelsey (1991) were more successful and felt less anxiety when their dogs were present than when a close friend was with them. This finding was attributed to the feeling of unconditional support not always found through friends (Allen et al., 1991). Other benefits from human-animal interactions are a reduction in feelings of loneliness and isolation, an increase in social interaction and emotional support, greater opportunities to experience joy, laughter and leisure, an increased ability to empathize with others, and promotion of nurturing skills (Fine, 2003; Steffens & Bergler, 1988). The psychological benefits of pet ownership have even been recognized by courts around the country as lawyers argue that under 1988 amendments to the Federal Fair Housing Act, landlords and co-op boards must allow tenants with mental/emotional disabilities to keep pets who act as emotional support animals (Rich, 2003).

Pet ownership has also shown an impact on depression levels in persons with serious medical conditions such as AIDS (Siegal, 1993). The study led by Siegal (1993) found that in a sample of 1,872 men with AIDS, depression levels were higher among those with few confidants. But persons with AIDS who owned pets reported less depression than those who did not. It is evident that the animals played an important role in the lives of their human companions, and at times they acted as important elements in social support systems. For example, Alan (not his real name), a young man living with AIDS, shared how important his pets were in enhancing his quality of life. He described feeling spiritually connected to his two cats, and he felt they acted intuitively to his needs. When he was feeling sad or lonely, they were constantly at his side and encouraging his attention. He strongly believed that the process of taking care of the cats, petting them and even singing to them, helped him redirect his attention from focusing on his own struggles and anxiety.

Finally, it may be helpful to review the model Gorczyca, Fine, and Spain (2000) developed to explain how the companionship of animals is critical for persons with AIDS and other chronic illnesses. The authors adapted Bronfenbrenner's ecosystem social support model to explain how animals make considerable contributions to the lives of persons with chronic illnesses. The authors also explain the evolution and development of the nationwide community-based program Pets Are Wonderful Support (PAWS). Gorczyca, Fine, and Spain (2000) explained that the organization, founded in 1987, supports individuals with AIDS by helping them keep their companion animals as long as possible in mutually healthy environments. The organization provides numerous support options including veterinary care, education about preventing zoonoses (diseases that can be transmitted to humans by other vertebrate animals or shared by both these populations), pet food banks, foster care and adoption planning, in-home pet care, and if medically needed, animal transportation.

ANIMAL-ASSISTED INTERVENTIONS (AAI)

Numerous terms have been used to describe the phenomena of incorporating animals in working with humans. According to LaJoie (2003), over 12 different terms are in existence today to describe this form of therapy. Terms such as "pet therapy," "animal-facilitated counseling," "pet-mediated therapy," and "pet psychotherapy" have been commonly used interchangeably as descriptive terms. Nevertheless, the two most widely utilized terms are "animal-assisted therapy" and "animal-assisted activities." Both these alternatives could be classified under the rubric of animal-assisted interventions.

The Delta Society's *Standards of Practice for Animal Assisted Therapy* (1996) defines animal-assisted therapy (AAT) as an intervention with specified goals and objectives delivered by a health or human service professional with specialized expertise in using an animal as an integral part of treatment. Whether provided in a group or individual setting, Delta Society reports that AAT promotes improvement in physical, social, emotional, and/or cognitive functioning. To help a client deal with issues of touch, a therapist may use the holding of a rabbit as a strategy to open a discussion with the child.

In contrast, animal-assisted activities (AAA) occur when specially trained professionals, paraprofessionals, or volunteers accompanied by animals interact with people in a variety of environments (Delta Society, 1996). In AAA, the same activity can be repeated for many different people or groups of people, the interventions are not part of a specific treatment plan and are not designed to address a specific emotional or medical condition, and detailed documentation does not occur. The familiar sight of volunteers taking their pets to visit patients at an assisted living facility meets the criteria for AAA.

THE HISTORY OF ANIMAL-ASSISTED THERAPY

The unique bond between humans and animals and its powerful impact on human well-being has been documented over hundreds of years. One of the earliest theories regarding the benefits of incorporating animals into the therapeutic process occurred at the York Retreat in England. Fine et al. (1996) reported that the Quakers established the retreat in 1792 to serve patients with various mental illnesses. Documents from the retreat identified the staff's belief that having animals on the grounds enhanced patients' morale and behavior. Historically, many others, including Florence Nightingale, have noted the value of incorporating animals as an aspect of the rehabilitation process. In *Notes on Nursing,* Nightingale (1860) strongly argued that a small pet animal was an excellent companion for the sick. Her impressions, similar to the Quakers, seemed to accurately portray how animals could contribute to the physical and mental health of individuals (Fine, 2002).

Published in 1944, Bossard's paper addressed the therapeutic value of dog ownership and the important role domestic animals play in family systems and in enhancing the emotional well-being of family members. In response to a later article by Bossard (1950) titled "I Wrote About Dogs," 1,033 letters were received asking for reprints or referring to his original article. Bossard concluded that,

> The responses to the original publication of the article were so frank, so spontaneous and from such a large segment of the population representing such a wide range of social strata, as to leave no doubt that the love of animals by humans is one of the

universals in existence of both. Household pets are an integral part of family life; they must be considered as a basic implement in mental hygiene. (p. 408)

In the early 1960s, child psychologist Boris Levinson became the leading disciple for the therapeutic value of utilizing animals in therapeutic settings after discovering that when his dog Jingles was left with a particularly noncommunicative child client, the child began engaging in a deep conversation and interacting with the friendly pup (Gonski, 1985; Mason & Hagan, 1999; Reichert, 1998). Levinson's promotion of "pet therapy" was met with cynicism and disdain by his professional audience. Despite the skepticism he encountered, Levinson (1970) further advocated that companion animals might serve not only as a means of reaching emotionally disturbed children, but also as an asset in the healthy development of children (1970).

Fine (2002) pointed out that a meeting titled *"Health Benefits of Pets,"* sponsored by the National Institutes of Health in September 1987, had a tremendous impact on showcasing the value of the human/ animal bond. The proceedings emphasized scientific evidence clearly demonstrating the physical and emotional benefits of pet ownership. In addition, the scholars also highlighted the importance of studying the relationships and attachments to animals as valuable emotional alternatives to those who were vulnerable to loneliness (e.g., the elderly and isolated children). This meeting has been a catalyst for the development of numerous animal visiting programs sponsored by the various humane societies for residents in long-term facilities.

ANIMAL-ASSISTED THERAPY IN PSYCHOTHERAPY

There are several basic tenets to consider when incorporating animals into therapeutic practice. Fine (2003) strongly encourages clinicians to utilize a simple problem-solving approach as they begin to plan AAT therapeutic interventions with their patients. Therapists should consider the following three questions:

1. What benefits can AAT provide this client?
2. How can AAT strategies be incorporated within the planned intervention?
3. How will I need to adapt my approach to incorporate AAT?

The following section briefly describes basic strategies that can also be considered when incorporating AAT into clinical practice. This will be followed by more in-depth options.

Foundation 1: Animals Acting As a Social Lubricant

Animals can act as a social lubricant in a variety of settings. They can effectively ease the stress of the initial phase of therapy, act as a link in conversation between therapist and client, and help establish trust and rapport between patient and clinician. The mere presence of an animal can also give clients a sense of comfort, which further promotes rapport in the therapeutic relationship. A calm animal may also act as a signal of a safe environment. Since clients often view animals as an extension of the therapist, an animal may ease tension and act as an icebreaker when greeting clients with warmth and enthusiasm.

The case of Sarah illustrates the concept of the animal as a social lubricant (Fine, 2004). When the therapist first met Sarah (not her real name), a 14-year-old teen, she had a baseball cap pulled low on her head and was using the brim of the cap to cover her eyes. Sarah was referred for psychotherapy by her school due to the possibility of depression and suicidal ideation. At the first meeting, she barely responded, her voice was hardly above a whisper. During the first visit, Hart, the therapist's black Labrador "co-therapist," walked quietly to Sarah's side and sat close to her chair. At that meeting, Hart simply sat by Sarah in the waiting room, ready to be petted if Sarah felt like it. Sarah did not have an obvious reaction to Hart's appearance. But after a few seconds, Sarah reached out and began stroking Hart's head. She petted the dog without much show of emotion, and initially avoided looking at her therapist by petting Hart. Yet, it was obvious that her trembling decreased; the physical contact with Hart seemed to help ease the tension and anxiety she was feeling.

Sarah and the therapist spent the first three sessions getting acquainted. The sessions always started in the waiting room—Sarah sitting huddled in one of the chairs, the brim of her cap over her eyes. She continued to speak very quietly and at times seemed to shiver with fear. The only time she seemed to relax was when she touched Hart. However, progress was slow with Sarah. In the first few visits, she primarily petted Hart and listened to the therapist, but divulged little.

It felt as if the client and therapist were treading water, but he didn't want to push her; his initial goal was to simply to build a relationship with this seriously withdrawn girl—a relationship she could trust and eventually learn from.

Over the course of the initial visits, the therapist managed to learn a little more about Sarah. Sarah told him that she had no real friends and that she felt like an outcast. Many of her peers ignored her because they thought she was different and they interpreted her fear as aloofness. She was afraid to speak up, afraid to approach others; she was pretty much just afraid. Sarah also began to report that she felt very anxious in public settings, which she tried to avoid. She suffered tremendous anxiety in school and reported feeling depressed and experiencing panic attacks. During the third session, Sarah finally revealed that over the past few months she begun to cut herself, initially on her arm with a pin and then with a sharp razor. She kept her wounds hidden from everyone, but for some reason she was now ready to reveal her secret.

As she sat and talked with her therapist, Hart, who seemed more alert than usual to Sarah's every move, sat close by her chair. At one point in the session, Sarah's reserve finally crumbled. Pushing up her left sleeve, she showed both Hart and her therapist her scars. As she lowered her arm, Sarah noticed that Hart's eyes were fixed on her arm. At that moment, Hart lifted her gaze and connected with Sarah. Hart then looked over at the therapist. With a puzzled expression on her face, Hart looked back to Sarah. Hart then lowered her head and began softly and tenderly licking the healed wounds. For a startled moment, Sarah sat still and then she bent over Hart and held her close.

Although no words were spoken, the therapist could tell that some barrier had fallen for Sarah. It was as if she said, "Now that we all know about this, we can talk about it and I can learn to never do this again." From that point on, there was accelerated progress. Sarah's improvement was remarkable. Integrated strongly within the therapeutic intervention was her relationship with Hart. Through Hart's support, she began to not only open up, but also to become more willing to follow the therapeutic regime and work on expressing herself, venturing out, and interacting with others as well as discarding her emotional shell.

Foundation 2: A Catalyst for Emotion

For many clients, the mere presence of an animal in a therapeutic setting can stir emotions. Simply interacting with an animal in a therapeutic setting can lighten the mood and lead to smiling and laughter. Animals also can display emotions and behavior that may not be professionally appropriate for therapists to display. For example, the animal might climb into a client's lap or sit calmly while the client pets him. Holding or petting an animal may soothe clients and help them feel calm when exploring difficult emotions in treatment that might be overwhelming without this valuable therapeutic touch. The presence of a trusted animal in therapy may also lend comfort and stability to the environment when a therapist must confront a client.

Foundation 3: Adjuncts to Clinicians

Having an animal in therapy may prove to be a catalyst for discussion, especially when clients have commonalities with animals. Some patients may see similarities between their own emotions and the perceived emotions expressed by an animal, such as shyness or fear. For example, children who have been abused or neglected may feel comfortable relating to an animal which was also abused or abandoned, and this may lead to sharing about their own abuse or abuse of a family member or pet they have witnessed.

This was often illustrated during animal-assisted group play-therapy sessions with children at a domestic violence crisis center, in which animals from the local humane society's AAT program were incorporated into treatment as a catalyst for discussion about the children's exposure to domestic violence. It should be noted that the animals utilized in treatment were temperament-tested, trained for interaction as therapy pets, and rehabilitated if they had experienced abuse. These sessions began with instruction from a humane society representative about how to approach and handle the pets, which often included a dog with only one eye. Then, the pets were introduced to the children and the pets' stories were told, including a description of abuse and/or abandonment the pet(s) had suffered (without being graphic and frightening). As children held or petted the animals, they often made unsolicited empathetic responses about the animals' abuse, such as "poor little puppy—I bet you sure are glad you have a safe home now." Children often shared their sadness due to memories of losing an animal either due to a natural death or because the pet was killed or removed from the home by an abusive parent. They also shared memories of abuse they witnessed, and the resulting fear they suffered and still carried with them. Some felt guilty that they couldn't protect their family members from abuse. Others expressed sadness at being separated from, or in their perception abandoned by, their abusive parent. Group facilitators then addressed the children's grief, fear, and related emotions in a nonthreatening setting, where petting the dog or cat seemed to lessen their anxiety and allowed them to be more open about emotions that they believed they shared with the abused or abandoned animals.

Fine (2004) also reported how he has incorporated a few animals who have been victims of violence to help his young clients express their feelings. The two most effective animals he has integrated into treatment are a bearded dragon (a type of lizard) named Spikey, who was injured at a pet store and lost part of her tail, and Fine's first therapy dog named Puppy, who came into the therapist's life when the dog escaped from her previous abusive history. Puppy was found running on the streets, and it was easy to tell she was an abused and neglected dog. She was scared of human touch and was missing a few of her teeth. It took some time for her to become more at ease with human contact. Nevertheless, over a little time and with kindness, love, and lots of attention, Puppy became more trusting. Puppy seemed to thrive with the attention; she soon loved being around people. After careful training and testing, Puppy was ready to become a therapy dog. Clients have found her presence very relaxing. On occasion, the therapist has discussed Puppy's past with clients who have experienced abuse as a method for helping clients to understand how one can work through his or her past. Puppy's presence in these instances has not only relaxed clients, but has also acted as a catalyst to discuss the events of the past and ways to overcome trauma.

Animals in therapeutic settings may also serve as vicarious role models. The clinician's interaction with animals may elicit comparisons with clients' own relationships, which the clinician can use for increasing insight or for teaching. For example, when boundaries are set with animals, clinicians can demonstrate limit setting as a valuable teaching tool for clients. A therapist might explain that just as a therapy animal must learn to follow direction and interact appropriately with participants in order for therapy sessions to be safe and enjoyable, it is important for child clients to follow their teacher's instructions and interact appropriately with classmates so the classroom will be a safe and enjoyable learning environment.

Foundation 4: The Therapeutic Environment— Animals As an Aspect of Milieu Therapy

Animals can be a valuable contribution to the therapeutic environment by helping to create a setting that is perceived as friendly and comfortable to clients. Langs (1979) suggests that the development of an effective therapeutic alliance may begin with the creation of a welcoming therapeutic environment. Fine (2000) reported that his clients appeared more willing to engage and more at ease as a consequence of the warmth radiated by his therapy animals.

INTEGRATING AAT INTO PSYCHOTHERAPY PRACTICE

As with any newly learned modality, therapists are advised to use caution and only incorporate approaches in which they have training and expertise. It is imperative for therapists to keep clear records and documentation. Fine (2003) also strongly suggests that the purpose of AAT be discussed with the client to determine whether any reservations exist. A signed letter of agreement to engage in therapy utilizing animals is also advised.

There are numerous options for incorporating animals into therapeutic interventions. For example, using metaphors and stories incorporating animals is an appropriate extension to AAT. Imagery generated from animal-related metaphors used in therapy can help a client uncover specific emotions or patterns. A client who feels overwhelmed might identify with a wish to fly freely with the birds, while someone trapped in a bad relationship may feel like a caged tiger, or a client emerging from a depressive episode might liken their metamorphosis to that of a caterpillar becoming a butterfly. The various metaphors used by therapists and clients help to clarify and accentuate their current state or their progress in treatment. Stories portraying the challenges, obstacles, and successes that animals experience and overcome may be applied therapeutically to help clients see the world or the struggles they face from a different perspective.

For example, a therapist who works at a residential treatment center for mothers recovering from substance abuse and their children keeps a picture of her dog Sam in her office and tells stories about him in therapy sessions with children. When she meets new child clients, the therapist explains that when Sam first came from the animal shelter to live with her, he was very afraid and didn't trust anyone. But over time, Sam saw that he was safe and well cared for in his new home, and he was not afraid any more. Sam's story helps normalize the children's fear of being in a new home surrounded by people they don't know or trust, and it gives them hope that just as Sam did, they too will overcome their fear and feel safe and happy in their new home.

Other unique options that lend themselves quite well with traditional AAT are reflective writings about the animals' and the patients' lives, therapeutic walks with the animals, as well as encouraging some clients to volunteer to work with animals.

Fine (2000) has also found role-playing to be a viable approach to AAT for work with children. Role-playing is especially valuable in encouraging children to reveal private symbols and thoughts. Children may feel more comfortable projecting their own emotions onto a therapy animal without having to take responsibility for what has been said. For example, a child who has been sexually abused or witnessed family violence might find it less intimidating to describe the fear, anger, and sadness a therapy animal might feel in that situation than to accept and describe his or her own personal terror (Reichert, 1998). By placing the focus of sessions on the therapy pet and its emotions rather than the client or the problem that led to the clinician's involvement, children may also let their guard down enough to begin opening up first to the nonthreatening pet, then to the therapist as an extension of the pet (Gonski, 1985).

Animal-assisted therapy may also be applied in clinical practice from a life stage perspective. As people progress through developmental stages, a variety of specific psychosocial challenges are faced, and AAT may effectively be incorporated into practice to help clients address these challenges. For example, when working with young children, an animal may provide a sense of unconditional love, fulfilling the most basic of developmental needs. Being able to master and guide an animal's behavior during sessions and learning the importance of behavior modification may promote a valuable sense of competence for children. Following Winnicott's theory of "the good enough parent," children may be able to experience a form of re-parenting through a close emotional and tactile relationship with an animal companion (Melson, 2001). Adolescents may feel less defensive when they are able to receive comfort from or project emotions onto an animal present in therapeutic settings, and they may be able to identify with some of the animal's characteristics such as playfulness or devotion. A therapy animal may serve as an impetus for discussions about relationship issues with adult clients, including having or raising children. Among single individuals, whether widowed, divorced, or never married, and childless couples or empty nesters, companion animals may serve as significant emotional substitutes for children or spouses. Finally, elderly clients may find that a therapy animal triggers memories from the past, which may help them reconnect to their life history and address unresolved issues from their past in therapy. The presence of an animal in the lives of elderly clients may also help clients feel useful and valued, or may help them deal with feelings of despair that may be an issue late in life.

Incorporating animals into therapy may also help clients manifest important issues that may otherwise not be addressed in treatment (Mason & Hagan, 1999; Sable, 1995). A study by Mason and Hagan (1999) reported a number of cases in which this occurrence was observed. In one case the therapy pet became a target of projection for the client's own feelings of anger. Through the therapeutic process (and under close supervision) the client worked through his anger and came to build a positive relationship with the pet. Other cases focused on in the study reported a theme of jealousy, when clients were upset that a pet was present in sessions because they wanted 100 percent of the therapist's attention. Once again, most clients were able to examine their true feelings of poor self-esteem and successfully work through this issue with the therapy pet present. Other clinicians interviewed for this study agreed that animal-assisted therapy appeared to be effective in working with clients diagnosed with anxiety disorders due to the calming effect of the therapy pet's presence in sessions.

The death of a beloved pet may be a traumatic loss experienced by clients, especially those who have difficulty with building human attachments and instead rely on their animal companion as their primary source of emotional support (Levinson, 1984; Sable, 1995). By helping clients process their grief at the loss of a pet, therapists may also help clients access previously unresolved feelings of loss. These feelings may be productively addressed in a therapeutic setting with an animal companion present to offer comfort and support (Levinson, 1984; Butler & Lagoni, 1996). When a child client is faced with the death of a pet, therapists have an opportunity to work with the family to ensure that the child is encouraged to grieve the loss while also learning appropriate life-lessons about death. Whether the loss of a pet is expected or unexpected, children benefit from honest, developmentally appropriate information about the death of a companion animal that avoids the use of euphemisms about death, along with involvement in advance of, during, and following the loss (Butler & Lagoni, 1996). Such involvement may include explaining a pet's illness to a child, including a child in discussions about when a terminally ill animal will be euthanized, and encouraging a child to participate in some form of memorial ceremony following the animal's death. Children may also need guidance to appropriately grieve the loss of a therapy animal when AAT concludes. Helping child clients prepare for closure in this relationship may better prepare them for future inevitable partings from other loved ones such as teachers, friends, or family members. Whatever the circumstances leading to the loss of a relationship with a beloved pet, children may benefit from receiving a transitional object such as a photograph of the child and pet together, a paw print from the pet, or the pet's favorite toy (Butler & Lagoni, 1996).

Some clients may initially be fearful of cats or dogs in a therapeutic setting. A clinician may be able to help these clients examine the underlying source of this fear, and of other fears, and determine whether or not their fear is rational. For example, some fears may be unfounded (e.g., a client's parent was afraid of dogs) or may stem from a remote incident that was perceived as more threatening than it actually was (e.g., a hyperactive dog knocked over and frightened a client when he or she was a toddler) (Gonski, 1985; Mason & Hagan, 1999). Clients may process how unfounded fears led to limitations in their lives. Many clients find that overcoming their fear of animals and eventually enjoying interaction with a therapy pet gives them a sense of accomplishment and pride, and that this successful experience of overcoming fear could be transferred to other areas of their lives (Mason & Hagan, 1999). In order to encourage a hesitant client to include a pet in the problem-solving process, it may be helpful during an early therapy session to introduce a photograph of the therapy pet and discuss the client's past animal-related experiences (Gonski, 1985). However, if a client declines to work with a pet co-facilitator, AAT should not be attempted (Gonski, 1985; Mason & Hagan, 1999).

Household pets may be a powerful indicator of domestic violence or abuse in a family unit. A number of studies show that domestic violence victims often report that their abuser had also injured or killed a pet, and anecdotal evidence suggests that animal abuse may indicate higher lethality in domestic violence relationships (Ascione, 1998; Ascione, Weber, & Wood, 1997; Flynn, 2000; Quinn, 2000). In addition, children who abuse animals may be imitating family violence or exerting control over a less powerful creature due to physical abuse they themselves are suffering (Flynn, 2000; Quinn, 2000). Because children are often more open about abuse that has occurred to a pet than about violence directed toward themselves or a family member, engaging children in a relationship with a therapy pet and asking children about their own pets may help children feel more comfortable in sharing facts about family violence (Quinn, 2000).

When appropriate, a therapist may also recommend a pet for clients. However, when recommending a pet, therapists must consider the challenges associated with companion animals and appropriately educate clients about pet care. Among the greatest challenge that may not be fully anticipated by perspective pet owners is the financial cost of pet ownership. The average dog-owning U.S. household visited their veterinarian two times a year with an annual expenditure of close to $200 a year (Gonzalez, 2002). Additional expenses for food, licensing, training, grooming, toys, and other supplies can also be substantial. Clients should be advised to thoroughly consider how much they can afford and are willing to spend on a pet. Consideration should also be given to the level of commitment clients are willing to make to a pet, as pets' average life spans vary from as little as 1.5 years for a mouse (The Humane Society, 2004b) to 50 years or more for a large bird like an African Gray Parrot (The Humane Society, 2004a). The amount of time and attention needed by pets varies by species and breed as well. Clearly, the decision to add a pet to a household requires careful consideration, and therapists who recommend pets to their clients hold an ethical responsibility to empower clients to make a pet acquisition that is beneficial to both clients and companion animals.

THE NEED FOR FURTHER RESEARCH

Although significant strides have been made in exploring the value of animal/human relationships, it is important to point out that there continues to be limited empirical support and research validating the overall effectiveness of AAT/AAA (Fine, 2000, 2002, 2003). Many researchers and scholars (Katcher, 2000) note that although the utilization of animals may be highly appealing, the evidence that a patient has enjoyed an interaction with an animal does not imply that the procedure is therapeutic. It appears that the biggest challenge facing advocates of AAT who claim that it improves outcomes is the need for documentation and scientific evidence (Voelker, 1995). Fine (2000) recommends demystifying AAT and encourages researchers from various academic backgrounds to institute best practice studies demonstrating AAT's efficacy with a wide range of special populations. Furthermore, there needs to be a more appropriate bridge between clinical practice and best practice research. Clinicians are encouraged to clearly document their approaches and pay close attention to the need for program evaluation. These developments may help researchers evaluate protocols and research techniques and best practice approaches with specific populations. A more thorough investigation of all of these efforts should assist the scientific community with the needed research priorities. As the field of AAT becomes more refined, it would be helpful for clinicians to follow prescribed procedures that have been empirically found to be more reliable and effective with specific populations. For example, further study may help determine whether specific AAT strategies are more valuable when working with children in outpatient treatment who are shy versus elderly populations in long-term residential settings.

GUIDELINES FOR DEVELOPING AN AAT PROGRAM

Mallon, Ross, and Ross (2000) and Fine and Stein (2003) provided several guidelines for developing and designing AAT programs. They concur in urging clinicians to obtain appropriate AAT training. The Delta Society's Pet Partner Program strongly advocates that clinicians must have training on techniques of AAT and AAA. Therapists should also contact their insurance carrier to notify the carrier that AAT is being practiced, to assess coverage and address any questions the carrier may have. Requirements and coverage vary among insurers, and some may require a special binder for practicing AAT.

In addition, all animals must be screened for their temperament to make sure they are appropriate candidates for AAT. While dogs and cats tend to be the most widely utilized therapy animals, other pets such as rabbits, bearded dragons, guinea pigs, birds, and others have successfully been utilized in AAT. Clinicians are encouraged to utilize the standards of practice guidelines suggested by the Delta Society or Therapy Dogs International. When using a dog in a clinical practice, the Canine Good Citizens Test (one of many dog obedience tests) should be mastered. While some of the following basic characteristics apply most directly to dogs, they should be present to some degree in therapy animals:

- Social and friendly (enjoy human interaction)
- Calm and gentle
- Good temperament
- Playful
- Able to handle unusual sights, sounds, and smells
- Well-mannered
- Familiar with basic obedience
- Able to regain self-control after play or excitement
- Able to sit quietly for extended periods
- All animals should be exposed to a variety of people, situations, and environments so they can handle novel situations.
- Able to manage anxiety when exposed to highly charged emotional people and situations
- Able to navigate through crowded environments
- Attentive to the therapist
- Mature (e.g., dogs should be at least 18 months of age)

Finally, it is critical that all clients should be interviewed to assess their comfort level with various animals, specific allergies, fears of animals and, if relevant, past abusive behavior toward animals. Each of these points may represent a contraindication for AAT.

ANIMAL WELFARE

Fine, Serpell, and Hines (2001) discuss ethical questions about the use of animals as therapeutic aides that arise out of tension between interests. While the therapeutic advantages of AAT to humans may be obvious, the benefits to the animals utilized in therapy are by no means always self-evident. AAA/T has experienced explosive growth within the past two decades, and in many cases inferred standards have been set in the absence of any systematic or empirical evaluation of the potential risks to animals. Indeed, the use of animals for animal-assisted activities and therapy poses a unique set of stresses and strains on animals that the "industry" is only just beginning to acknowledge, which may unfortunately lead to unintentional maltreatment of therapy animals. Ultimately, as practitioners, the safety of one's patient should be the highest priority. Nevertheless, it is vital that therapists entering AAT practice be fully aware of the considerations necessary to safeguard the animals' integrity and welfare. The following list developed by Serpell, Coppinger, and Fine (2000) represents some guidelines for clinicians to consider.

1. All animals must be kept free from abuse, discomfort, and distress.
2. Proper health care for the animal must be provided at all times. Animals must receive proper husbandry and have a proper diet.
3. All animals should have a quiet place where they can have time away from their work activities.
4. Interactions with clients must be structured as to maintain the animal's capacity to serve as a useful therapeutic agent.
5. Situations of abuse or stress for a therapy animal should never be allowed. As noted earlier, in the event where a client intentionally or unintentionally subjects a therapy animal to abuse,

the animal's needs must be considered and the interaction must
be discontinued.

6. As an animal ages, his/her schedule for therapeutic involvement will
have to be curtailed. Accommodations and plans must be considered. The transition into retirement may also be emotionally difficult
for the animal. Attention must also be given to this dimension.

CONCLUSION

As commonly quoted author Bern Williams once stated, "There is
no psychiatrist in the world like a puppy licking your face" (http://en
.thinkexist.com/quotes/bern_williams/). Incorporating animals into clinical settings represents a dynamic alternative for mental health provid-
ers involved in the treatment of children and adults in both outpatient
and institutional settings, and in individual or group therapy. Although
not a panacea, clinicians are encouraged to investigate the tremendous
potential value of this complementary therapy.

Animals need to be introduced into therapy with a well-thought-
out plan and integrated into a clinician's therapeutic approach. It is
imperative that committed therapists receive the appropriate training
to institute this form of treatment and that every precaution is made to
ensure the integrity and safety of both the clients and the animals.
When this thoughtful approach is followed, the unconditional positive regard conveyed by therapy animals may greatly contribute to
positive outcomes in clinical practice.

REFERENCES

Ainsworth, M. (1989). Attachment beyond infancy. *American Psychologist, 44,*
709-716.

Albert, A. & Bulcroft, K. (1988). Pets, families and the life course. *Journal of
Marriage and the Family, 50*(May), 543-552.

Allen, K. (2003). Are pets a healthy pleasure? The influence of pets on blood pressure. *Current Directions in Psychological Science,12*(6), 236-239.

Allen, K., Blascovich, J., Tomaka, & Kelsey, R. (1991). The presence of human
friends and pet dogs as moderators of autonomic responses to stress in women.
Journal of Personality and Social Psychology, 61(4), 582-589.

Archer, J. (1997). Why do people love their pets. *Evolution and Human Behavior,
18,* 237-259.

Ascione, F. (1998). Battered women's reports of their partners' and their children's cruelty to animals. *Journal of Emotional Abuse, 1.* Retrieved November 29, 2001, from www.vachss.com/guest_dispatches/ascione_3.html.

Ascione, F., Weber, C., & Wood, D. (1997). The abuse of animals and domestic violence: A national survey of shelters for women who are battered. *Society and Animals, 5*(3). Retrieved November 29, 2001, from http://www.vachss.com/guest_dispatches/ascione_1.html.

Barba, B.E. (1995). A critical review of research on the human/companion animal relationship: 1988 to 1993. *Anthrozoos, 8,* 9-15.

Bossard, J. (1944). The mental hygiene of owning a dog. *Mental Hygiene, 28,* 408-413.

Bossard, J. (1950). I wrote about dogs. *Mental Hygiene, 34,* 345-349.

Bowlby, J. (1969). Disruption of affectional bonds and its effects on behavior. *Canada's Mental Health Supplement, 69,* 1-17.

Bowlby, J. (1980). *Attachment and loss.* New York: Basic Books.

Butler, C. & Lagoni, L. (1996). Children and pet loss. In C. Coor, & D. Corr, (Eds.), *Handbook of childhood death and bereavement.* New York: Springer Publishing Company.

Delta Society. (1996). Standards of practice in animal-assisted activities and therapy.

Fine, A.H. (2000). Animals and therapists: Incorporating animals in outpatient psychotherapy. In A. Fine (Ed.), *Handbook on animal assisted therapy: Theoretical foundations and guidelines for practice* (pp. 179-211). San Diego: Academic Press.

Fine, A.H. (2002). Animal assisted therapy. In M. Hersen & W. Sledge (Eds.), *Encyclopedia of psychotherapy* (pp. 49-55). New York: Elsevier Science.

Fine, A.H. (2003). Animal Assisted Therapy and Clinical Practice. Psycho legal Associates CEU meeting, November, 1, Seattle, WA.

Fine, A.H. (2004). Submitted for publication. Afternoons with puppy: A therapist, his therapy animals and life changes.

Fine, A.H., Lee, J., Zapf, S., Kirwin, S., & Henderson, K. (1996). Broadening the impact of services and recreational therapies. In A. Fine & N. Fine (Eds.) *Therapeutic recreation and exceptional children* (2nd ed.) (pp. 53-86). Springfield, IL: Charles C Thomas.

Fine, A.H., Serpell, J., & Hines, L. (2001). *The welfare of assistance and therapy animals: An ethical commentary.* International Conference on the Human Animal Bond, Rio, Brazil, September, 14.

Fine, A.H. & Stein, L. (2003). Animal assisted therapy and clinical practice. Psycho legal Associates CEU meeting, October, 25, Pasadena, CA.

Flynn, C. (2000). Why family professionals can no longer ignore violence toward animals. *Family Relations, 49,* 87-95.

Friedman, E., Katcher, A.H., Lynch, J.J., & Thomas, S.A. (1980). Animal companions and one-year survival of patients after discharge from a coronary care unit. *Public Health Reports, 95,* 301-312.

Friedman, E., Katcher, A.H., Thomas, S., Lynch, J.J., & Messant, P. (1983). Social Interaction and blood pressure: Influence of animal companions. *Journal of Nervous and Mental Disease, 171,* 461-465.

Garrity, T. & Stallones, L. (1998). Effects of pet contact on human well being. In C. Wilson & D. Turner (Eds.), *Companion animals in human health* (pp. 3-22). Thousand Oaks, CA: Sage Publishers.

Gonski, Y. (1985). The therapeutic utilization of canines in a child welfare setting. *Child & Adolescent Social Work Journal, 2*(2), 93-105.

Gonzalez, M. (2002). *US Pet ownership and demographic sourcebook: Vet market statistics.* Schaumburg, IL: AVMA.

Gorczyca, K., Fine, A.H., & Spain, C.V. (2000). History, theory and development of human-animal support services for people with AIDS and other chronic/terminal illnesses. In A. Fine (Ed.), *Handbook on animal assisted therapy: Theoretical foundations and guidelines for practice* (pp. 253-302), San Diego: Academic Press.

Gunter, B. (1999). *Pets and people: The psychology of pet ownership.* London: Whurr Publishers Ltd.

Hart, L.A. (1993). Companion animals throughout the human life cycle: The contributions of Aline and Robert Kidd. *Anthrozoös, 6,* 148-153.

Hirsch-Pasek, K. & Treiman, R. (1982). Doggerel: Motherese in a new context. *Journal of Child Language, 9,* 229-237.

The Humane Society of the United States. (2004a). Birds as pets. Retrieved February 15, 2004, from www.hsus.org/ace/11765?pg=1.

The Humane Society of the United States. (2004b). Mouse. Retrieved February 15, 2004, from www.hsus.org/ace/12265.

Hunt, S., Hart, L.A, & Gomulkiewicz, R. (1992). Role of small animals in social interaction between strangers. *Journal of Social Psychology, 133,* 245-256.

Katcher, A.H. (2000). Animal assisted therapy and the study of human-animal relationships: Discipline or bondage? Context or transitional object? In A. Fine (Ed.), *Handbook on animal assisted therapy: Theoretical foundations and guidelines for practice* (pp. 461-473). San Diego, CA: Academic Press.

LaJoie, K.R. (2003). An evaluation of the effectiveness of using animals in therapy. Unpublished doctoral dissertation, Spalding University, Louisville, KY. (University Microfilms, No. 3077675).

Langs, R. (1979). *The therapeutic environment.* New York: Jason Aronson.

Lee, D. (1984). Companion animals in institutions. In P. Arkow (Ed.), *Dynamic relationships in practice: Animals in the helping professions* (pp. 237-256). Alameda, CA: Latham Foundation.

Levinson, B.M. (1970). Pets, child development and mental illness. *Journal of the American Veterinary Medical Association, 157,* 1759-1766.

Levinson, B.M. (1984). Grief at the loss of a pet. In W. Kay, H. Nieburg, A. Kutscher, R. Grey, & C. Fudin, (Eds.), *Pet loss and human bereavement.* Ames, IA: The Iowa State University Press.

Lynch, J. & McCarthy, J. (1969). Social responding dogs: Heart rate changes to a person. *Psychophysiology, 5*(4), 389-393.

Mallon, G., Ross, S., & Ross, L. (2000). Designing and implementing animal assisted therapy programs in health and mental health organizations. In A. Fine (Ed.), *Handbook on animal assisted therapy: Theoretical foundations and guidelines for practice.* (pp. 115-127), San Diego, CA: Academic Press.

Mason, M. & Hagen, C. (1999). Pet-assisted psychotherapy. *Psychological Reports, 84*(3), 1235-1245.

McNicholas, J. & Collis, G. (1995). The end of the relationship: Coping with pet loss. In I. Robinson (Ed.), *The Waltham book of human-animal interaction: Benefits and responsibilities of pet ownership* (pp.127-143). Oxford: Pergamon.

Melson, G. (2001). *Why the wild things are: Animals in the lives of children.* Cambridge, MA: Harvard University Press.

Messant, P. (1984). Correlates and effects of pet ownership. In E. Anderson, B. Hart, & L. Hart (Eds.), *The pet connection: Its influence on our health and quality of life* (pp. 331-340). Minneapolis, MN: University of Minnesota.

Montague, J. (1995). Continuing care—Back to the garden. *Hospitals and Health Networks, 69*(17), 58.

Mugford & M'Cominsky, J. (1975). Some recent work on the psychotherapeutic value of cage birds with old people. In R.S. Anderson (Ed.), *Pet animals and society* (pp. 54-65). London: Bailliere-Tindall.

Muschel, U. (1985). Pet therapy with terminal cancer patients. *Social Casework: The Journal of Contemporary Social Work, 65,* 451-458.

Nightingale, F. (1860). *Notes on nursing.* New York: D. Appleton and Company.

Quinn, K. (2000). Animal abuse at early age linked to interpersonal violence. *The Brown University Child and Adolescent Behavior Letter, 16*(3). Retrieved November 26, 2001 from www.childresearch.net/cybrary/news/200003.html.

Raina, P., Waltner-Toews, B., Bonnett, B., Woodward, C., & Abernathy, T. (1999). Influence of companion animals on the physical and psychological health of older people. *Journal of American Geriatric Society, 47*(3), 323-329.

Reichert, E. (1998). Individual counseling for sexually abused children: A role for animals in storytelling. *Child and Adolescent Social Work Journal, 15*(3), 177-185.

Rich, M. (2003, June 26). Pet therapy sets landlords howling. *New York Times.*

Sable, P. (1995). Pets, attachment and well-being across the life cycle. *Social Work, 40*(3), 334-340.

Selby, L.A. & Rhoades, J.D. 1981. Attitudes of the public towards dogs and cats as companion animals. *Journal of Small Animal Practice, 22,* 129-37.

Serpell, J. Coppinger, R., & Fine, A. (2000). The welfare of assistance and therapy animals: An ethical comment. In A. Fine (Ed.), *Handbook on animal assisted therapy: Theoretical foundations and guidelines for practice* (pp. 415-430). San Diego,CA: Academic Press.

Siegel, J. (1993). Companion animals: In sickness and in health. *Journal of Social Issues, 49,* 157-167.

Steffens, M. & Bergler, R. (1988). Blind people and their dogs: An empirical study on changes in everyday life, in self-experience, and in communication. In C. Wilson & D. Turner (Eds.), *Companion animals and human health* (pp. 149-157). Thousand Oaks, CA: Sage Publishers.

Voelker, R. (1995). Puppy love can be therapeutic, too. *The Journal of the American Medical Association, 274,* 1897-1899.

Young, J. (2003). Creature comforts, fresh finds. *Richmond Times-Dispatch,* July 12, F3.

Zasloff, R. & Kidd, A. (1994). Attachment to feline companions. *Psychological Reports, 74,* 747-752.

Chapter 10

Touch Therapies

Anne L. Strozier
Catherine E. Randall
Erin Kuhn

Touch, outside the framework of psychotherapy, can be an easy and comforting way to communicate. Touching the soft curls of our school-bound kindergartener, embracing an elderly relative, or holding the hand of one's partner are all examples of warm and loving nonverbal expressions. Touch can explicitly express our caring feelings without saying a word.

Although touch therapies may not be prevalent in traditional psychotherapy, the use of touch is finding its place among other diverse forms of therapy. Therapists often use gentle touch to communicate empathy and trust. Many complementary therapies, especially those rooted in ancient history, embrace the benefits of touch, and incorporate it in their daily practice. These therapies include Reiki, therapeutic touch, and massage therapy and use touch to heal both the physical and energetic body.

This chapter includes theories, historical information, research, guidelines, and case examples in the following areas: touch in psychotherapy, Reiki, therapeutic touch, and massage therapy. In the first part of this chapter, we will discuss the use of touch in psychotherapy, the pros and cons, and brief case examples. In the second part of the chapter, we will describe several of the complementary touch therapies including Reiki, therapeutic touch, and massage therapy along with ethical and legal guidelines for touch therapy.

Introduction to Alternative and Complementary Therapies
doi:10.1300/5987_10

TOUCH IN PSYCHOTHERAPY

The use of touch with clients in psychotherapy is controversial. Some theorists believe that touch should never be used, while others hold that touch can enhance the therapeutic process. These disagreements concerning touch in therapy reflect early controversy that seems to have originated with Freud, who, himself, used touch in his early work with patients: "(Freud) used massage to the neck and head to facilitate emotional expression and age regression in his patients, while allowing them to touch him" (Kertay & Reviere, 1993, p. 33). But in his growing focus on transference and his belief that the therapist should be a "blank slate," Freud withdrew his support of the use of touch.

Sandor Ferenczi was the leading advocate of touch in the early days of psychoanalysis. While Freud and Ferenczi disagreed about many analytic techniques, Ferenczi (1993) viewed touch as an empathic response to the analysis and, one which incorporated a "language of tenderness and passion" (p. 156). Ferenczi further believed that the analyst risked repeating the patient's original trauma if he remained neutral and detached as recommended by Freud. This early dispute over touch continues: some theorists assert the great value of touch while others focus on its dangers and harmful effects.

Research: Positive Findings

Erik Erikson, Anna Freud, and other leading developmental and child psychologists note the importance of touch in "libidinizing the infant's body, developing body image, self-love and object love" (Kupfermann & Smaldino, 1987, p. 226). Other theorists observe that infants' failure to thrive may be attributed to a lack of touch (Field, Schanberg, & Scafidi, 1986). Wilson (1982) argues that because touch is such an important part of human development, it is important that we not dismiss its use as a psychotherapeutic intervention.

Some theorists believe that touch is so important that *not* using it in therapy may hinder clients. Older (1977) describes a client who interpreted her therapist's failure to touch her as evidence that she was untouchable and that her wish to be touched was a bad feeling. Fuchs (1975) also found that not touching "unwittingly, tends to reproduce the too cool, nonaffectional atmosphere which nourished the original neurosis . . . reinforce[ing] the very isolation from which the patient is so desperately trying to shake loose" (p. 169).

Several researchers described touch as being helpful in motivating clients to work hard in therapy (Jourard & Friedman, 1970; Pederson, 1973). Confirmation of this viewpoint came in Pattison's (1973) study of 20 female undergraduate clients, finding those who were touched engaged in more self-exploration. Touch has also been viewed as a way to "validate a client's existence as a human being who is connected with others" (Strozier, Krizek, & Sale, 2003).

Wilson (1982) suggested that the timing of touch in therapy is critical. She found that touch is most beneficial when the client is in the working phase of the relationship when trust has been established and the client is exploring new ways of coping.

Smith, Clance, and Imes (1998) provide the following positive experience from a client about touch in therapy:

> I can remember the first time that he touched me when I was very depressed. He came over to where I was sitting, and put his hands on my shoulders. And the respectfulness and the sensitivity with which he approached me—that in itself was very touching. He always allowed me freedom as to how much I would initiate touch, and those times when he would initiate would be times when I didn't feel connected. (p. 115)

Research: Negative Findings

On the other end of the spectrum, theorists express grave concerns about using touch in therapy. Some researchers even dictate a literal "hands-off" policy for psychotherapeutic work with clients (Durana, 1998). Major concerns include the ideas that touching clients may interfere with transference or that touch may foster dependency, gratify infantile needs, and allow other harms to the therapeutic relationship (Mintz, 1969; Wilson & Masson, 1986). Durana (1998) notes that touch in therapy may lead to power differentials, sexual victimization of the client, and complications in transference and countertransference processes (Durana, 1998). Kertay and Reviere (1993) report that "therapists who touched opposite sexed patients, but not same-sex patients, were at a significantly higher risk for sexual contact with patients" (p. 36). Strozier, Krizek, and Sale (2000) indicate that touch can cause "blurred boundaries, foster dependence, and interrupt the process of healing." Bacorn and Dixon (1984) caution that therapists may be using touch with clients only to ease their own anxiety. Ethics, regulations, and malpractice concerns also deter many therapists from using touch.

An area of great concern is the possible meaning that can be inferred from touch. Spotnitz (1972) warned that touch can have different meaning for different clients. He went on to say that clients who experience negative transference may respond to touch negatively by feeling disrespected, threatened, or even enraged. Older (1982) noted: "Touch a paranoid and risk losing a tooth, touch a seductress and risk losing your license. Touch a violent patient with a short fuse and risk losing everything" (p. 201).

If the research on using touch in therapy is mixed, views of experienced social workers are equally conflicted. Following are quotes about using touch in psychotherapy from experienced social workers from Strozier et al. (2000):

> I work in a psychiatric hospital with severely regressed extremely psychotic patients. Touch, therefore, is an important source of communication with them and a means of reaching out to establish a relationship.

> I found that a large number of clients didn't want me to touch them. Touch was confusing, not always perceived as supportive, and was too often a trigger for flashbacks of sexual abuse . . . Because of the unpredictable consequences, I am less likely to initiate touch when a client is experiencing an emotionally upsetting time during session.

> Touch done professionally can be a gesture of acceptance, comfort, and a model of a right way to touch someone without ulterior motives.

> I work with a large percentage of senior citizens in nursing homes where touch, i.e., of hands & maybe a pat on shoulder is extremely important. Majority of these clients have no visitors and the visit from their therapist is very important, primarily for those who are bed ridden.

I primarily work with young children who have been abused (physical and sexual). I feel it is important to teach/model that touch is positive.

Strongest reason I limit touch is to respect clients' personal/ physical boundaries.

Touch helps establish a relationship. It is, simply, Human.

Recent Research

Strozier et al. (2003) surveyed 91 "expert social workers" (defined as licensed clinical social workers who had been in practice for at least five years) about their use of touch with clients in psychotherapy. Findings indicate that a majority of social workers surveyed (95 percent) used some form of touch in their practice. The most frequently used types of touch were shaking of the hands or touching the client's arm, shoulder, or back. Social workers in this study indicated that they used touch generally when clients entered their offices or asked to be touched. These social workers were more likely to touch children and older clients, and those who were either physically ill or of the same gender. Curiously, social workers did not vary in their use of touch depending upon the theoretical orientation.

In a study by Milakovich (1998), he suggests that therapists who had supervisors who advocated the use of touch in therapy were significantly more likely to use touch in their own therapeutic practice. Results also showed that therapists who had personally experienced seven or more types of body therapies were significantly more likely to utilize touch in therapy. Furthermore, the belief that touch was a beneficial and necessary fundamental intervention for healing increased the likelihood that therapists would implement it in practice.

Guidelines for Using Touch in Psychotherapy

Minz outlined certain situations in which she believes touch may be appropriate: (1) as symbolic mothering at those times when the patient is incapable of verbal communication; (2) to communicate acceptance when the patient's self-loathing is overwhelming; (3) to strengthen or restore reality contact when it is threatened by anxiety; (4) as a means of controlled exploration of aggressive feelings, as for example, with the use of arm wrestling; and (5) when it is a natural expression of the therapist's feelings toward the client (Kertay & Reviere, 1993, p. 35).

A therapist trying to decide whether or not to touch a client may well remember the many physical, psychological, and emotional benefits that touch can bring to people in their everyday lives. The therapist may consider that touching a client in therapy will communicate affection, understanding, acceptance, and safety, and that touch can comfort the client who needs a sense of connection or emotional expression not possible through speech. At the same time, the therapist always needs to be aware of the fact that touch can also be a powerful means of triggering less positive responses in clients. Clients with a history of abuse or with repressed memories may feel frightened or victimized by even casual touch. Unwanted touch can severely damage the therapeutic relationship, in addition to being a clear violation of ethical guidelines. Any therapeutic approach involving touch must be accompanied by a clear understanding of the risks involved if the treatment is not approached with professionalism and skill.

Even if a therapist feels clear about the use of touch with a client, there still remains the potential for the client to misinterpret the therapist's intent or meaning.

> A female client misunderstood it (my touch of the client), and it contributed to eroticized transference issues getting out of hand. I went into therapy for five years afterward to deal with it. (Strozier, Krizek, & Sale, 2003)

In a Strozier, Krizek, and Sale (2003) study, results showed that although almost all of the social workers in the sample admitted to using touch in therapy, 82 percent reported they had no formal instruction as to its proper application. Overall, it seemed that intuition guided these professionals on the use of touch, and not education or theory.

> Touching, or not, or when to, grows out of the particulars of the work with a given client and I sense when it is the right thing to do. I tend to trust my instincts as I have had no negative outcomes and I am not much inclined to touch. So when I am I trust it as part of the "art" of counseling, arising form an intuitive sense of the moment. (Strozier et al., 2000)

Smith, Clance, and Imes (1998) pose three questions therapists should ask before they decide to implement touch into practice. Does the therapist have adequate theoretical and technical training? Does the therapist know the extent to which this practice is applicable to his or her client and its validity? Has the therapist had the proper amount of supervision to employ the strategy effectively?

The second question is referred to as the "ego-syntonic imperative." This question asks therapists whether a touch technique or use of touch is congruent with the therapist's style of therapy. This imperative also implies that the client or patient must use the therapist's method. Should the client wish to partake in a therapy with which the professional is not familiar, then the therapist should refer the client to the appropriate professional. The final question pertains to what the client's need is. Any and all touching should be done only in the client's best interests, working toward serving their therapeutic needs (Smith, Clance, & Imes, 1998).

Smith, Clance, and Imes (1998) quote one therapist's thoughts about when to touch and with whom:

> Generally, if I am feeling inclined to make physical contact with a client, I will share/talk about my sense of responsiveness to the client and will ask if my initiating contact fits with what the client is needing at the time. I will not make contact with a client unless I know it is what the client wants. The clients I do not initiate physical contact with are those who have some history of boundary violation (i.e., physical, sexual, emotional abuse) and/or have a tendency to oversexualize or be seductive, and/or have compromised/poorly differentiated ego boundaries. If, however, these clients initiate contact with me I do not reject their contact (unless it is really inappropriate . . . this has never been the case for me, however). (p. 101)

Hunter and Struve (1998) suggest a set of guidelines to govern decisions in therapeutic situations where touch is being considered. Several of these guidelines are:

- The client must be informed as to the purpose of touch.
- The boundaries governing touch should be explicitly delineated, communicated, and validated by the client.

- Therapists should seek written consent prior to the utilization of touch in therapy (although verbal confirmation is frequently used).
- The use of touch should clearly target the client's needs and welfare. If using touch serves more to satisfy the personal needs of the therapist than to address the presenting needs of the client, then such an intervention should not be implemented.
- The decision to use touch intervention should not be based on client characteristics preferred by and appealing to the therapist.
- The client should firmly comprehend the notions of empowerment and autonomy in a therapeutic setting. Clients must genuinely believe in the power of their choices to say "yes" or "no" to interventions such as touching without feeling those choices will be pressured or challenged by the therapist.
- It is important that rapport be established prior to using touch as a technique.
- It is essential that the therapist possesses an extensive knowledge base regarding the effectiveness of touch along with being trained adequately in its appropriate application.

REIKI

The history of Reiki has been passed down orally for thousands of years with different accounts of its history. Rand (1991) states that a form of energetic healing, often accompanied by sound, can be traced back to Buddhism thousands of years ago. However, the use of energy in healing has been described in many other ancient cultures. In China it is known as *ch'i* or *qui,* in India it is referred to as *prana,* in Native America it is *orenda* and in Hawaii it is *mana* (Stein, 1990). The practice of Reiki has its origins in Japan and had been long forgotten until Dr. Mikao Usui rediscovered this healing energy in the early 1900s. Dr. Usui is credited with documenting the symbols traditionally used in the treatment process and describing the process of attunement, which is the transmission of Reiki energy from teacher to student (Rand, 1991).

After Dr. Usui's death, Reiki continued to flourish in Japan under the guidance of Chujiro Hayashi, a protege of Dr. Usui. Dr. Hayashi opened the first Reiki clinic in Japan and is responsible for creating the standards for hand placement, the system of three degrees with the initiation procedures, and developing the Usui method of Reiki. Reiki became accessible to the West after a Japanese American woman from Hawaii, Hawayo Takata, received Reiki treatment for cancer while traveling to Japan. Convinced of its healing power, she not only became a Reiki master, but persuaded Dr. Hayashi to return with her to Hawaii and assist in establishing the first Reiki clinic in the United States. From 1970 until her death in 1980, Hawayo initiated 21 Reiki masters to carry on the tradition (Rand, 1991). Today Reiki is practiced in 48 countries and there are over 50,000 Reiki masters. As a result of this worldwide recognition, the International Reiki Association of Professionals (IARP) was established in 1997 to help propagate the practice. (IARP, 2003). Reiki, a form of bodywork, is based on the belief in a universal flow of healing energy (Rand, 1991). *Rei* and *Ki* are Japanese words that are generally translated to mean "universal life energy." This energy, or *Ki,* flows through and immediately around every living being. The field of energy around the body is called the aura, and energy flows from the aura into the body. The aura is sometimes referred to as a person's energy body, larger than and equally complex as the physical body. Energy flow in a person's aura can become disrupted even before the energy flow within the body is affected (Rand, 1991).

According to the principles of Reiki, when the healthy flow of energy in and around a body is blocked, it may result in physical pain or illness. These energy blocks in the body can be caused by emotional trauma, physical injury, and chronic illness. The energy block can cause a physiological response that increases stress and weakens the immune system, making it more difficult for the body to self-heal. Reiki can help relieve both the energy blocks and stress enabling the body to begin its natural recovery process.

Since *Ki* responds to a person's thoughts and feelings, the pattern of negative thoughts, conscious or unconscious, disrupt the flow of *Ki.* Reiki treatment targets these areas of disruption and channels positive energy to release negative, cognitive, and emotional blocks. A client often expresses strong emotional reactions during a Reiki treatment because of the buried and/or repressed emotions that the positive energy flow releases. It is believed that the body contains "memory" that the conscious mind rejects. This body memory is a function of *Ki* being disrupted by negative or painful thoughts, and causing physical pain or disease. Often Reiki will bring the repressed body memory into the client's conscious memory, forcing the client to confront difficult emotions (Rand, 1991).

Reiki can be practiced either in a traditional manner by placing hands on the client's clothed body or working in the client's aura which exists between one and four inches from the client. Treating the client's aura can be more powerful and is often most recommended, as this is the source of the healing energy before entering the body. The therapist's hands are placed on specific areas of the body, guided by either the client or the therapist's intuition. There is no right or wrong placements or positions in aura treatment, as the healing energy will flow throughout the client's body (Rand, 1991). For Reiki to be successful, both therapist and client must to be receptive to the idea of a healing energy and have a genuine desire to heal or be healed (IARP, 2005). A typical Reiki session starts with the clothed client lying supine on a flat surface. The practitioner silently acknowledges his or her intention to heal and requests the healing energy to flow, then suggests the client make a similar acknowledgment of receptivity. No meditation is necessary. Treatment begins with the therapist assessing or scanning the client's aura for areas that need attention. Over the course of one to one and a half hours, the therapist places his or her hands on or above places on the client's body that contain organs or chakra centers, the seven points on the energy body along the head and torso that correspond to endocrine glands in the physical body. The therapist generally addresses one place from three to ten minutes, depending on the perceived need for healing. At the end of the session, the therapist seals the client's energy field, either ritually or figuratively, essentially stopping the transfer of energy from therapist to client. Reiki can be administered as single treatments, such as surgery, or over multiple sessions to help with chronic pain.

The measurable effectiveness of Reiki lies in what the client may call a general feeling of well-being. Reiki reportedly induces the relaxation response, which is a physiological reaction manifesting lowered stress levels, deep calm breathing, and an increased immune response (IAPR, 2005). Stein (1990) stated a calming response in her experience of receiving Reiki:

As they worked, I felt great warmth moving through me, through all of my body, not only in the places being touched. At the end of it I felt fully calm, all physical and emotional tensions lifted. The feeling of being balanced and centered lasted for several days. (p. 53)

The effectiveness of Reiki in reducing stress from the body has inspired many health care professionals to not only support the use of Reiki in health care, but also to become trained Reiki masters. Dr. Philip Chan refers to Reiki as "a nontraditional bioenergetic system of stress relief" and by using multiple 15-minute-sessions has seen relief in headaches, muscle spasm, bursitis, dental pain, sinus congestion, and shingles (Chan, 2005, p. 1).

Reiki is also used by nurses to help facilitate the patient's healing process. Kathie Lipinski, RN, is a Reiki master and has used Reiki when inserting an IV, on incision wounds after surgery, and in labor and delivery. She is also a strong advocate for using Reiki as a self-care technique for busy nurses often stressed by demanding schedules (Lipinski, 2005).

Reiki is also making advances into hospital and clinic settings as well. According to Facilitating Awareness Through Empowerment (FATE), there are at least 10 hospitals in the United States that incorporate Reiki as part of their patient services. The Reiki clinic at the Tucson Medical Center in Arizona has a team of volunteer Reiki practitioners who provide treatment to patients in the hospital. What began as a trial basis in the oncology Cancer Care Unit has expanded to most areas in the hospital with a team of 20 Reiki volunteers. The California Pacific Medical Center, one of Northern California's largest hospitals, provides a wide range of complementary treatments. Dr. Cantwell, also a Reiki master, provides Reiki treatment and encourages patients to learn Reiki training for self-healing. Dr. Cantwell is currently conducting clinical research on Reiki to provide insurance companies with documented results of its effectiveness (Rand, 2005).

Training to become a Reiki practitioner involves learning from a Reiki master, one who has completed the master-level training. Rather than a traditional learning process, the ability to perform Reiki is transferred from master to student through attunements (Rand, 1991). The ability to channel Reiki is believed to be present within all people and requires only a connection to the source of this healing energy.

An "attunement" is the process in which the master transfers to the student the ability to channel the Reiki energy. During an attunement, the master makes changes in the student's energy pathways so that the student can access and channel *Ki*. Typically, between two and six attunements are required before the student is ready to perform Reiki treatments. The first and second classes of Reiki focus on teaching such things as hand positions, treatments, symbols, and distant healing. The advanced Reiki training teaches how to remove negative energy, and how to use crystals and stones. The last training class, Reiki III or master training, is a comprehensive review of previously learned material and advanced training through guided practice (Rand, 1991). The ability to perform Reiki is never lost, but continued attunements are encouraged to strengthen the practitioner's sensitivity to *Ki* (IARP, 2005).

THERAPEUTIC TOUCH

The term *therapeutic touch* was first coined by Dolores Krieger, PhD, RN, and Dora Kunz in the 1970s. Macrae (1987) provides a definition of this unconventional therapy as an act of healing or helping that is akin to the "ancient practice of laying-on of hands" (p. 3). However, it does not actually involve the "laying on of hands" because the practitioner works in the client's energy field, which exists a few inches from the body (Cohen, 1986).

> It just quiets. From the time that you're here doing the Therapeutic Touch, I am physically quiet and that quietness bleeds over into the rest of the day. It's been useful in the sense that it has calmed me. Giving me time. (Kiernan, 2002, p. 49)

Practitioners of therapeutic touch have traditionally been nurses or other professionals in health settings such as hospitals, clinics, and massage therapy offices. Therapeutic touch is taught in schools of medicine, nursing, and massage therapy, but is now more accessible to mental health professionals in the form of seminars and workshops. Courses generally consist of a foundation of the modality's concepts, philosophy, and basic practice. Therapists are then encouraged to seek mentorship with a skilled practitioner (Nurse Healers-Professional Associates International [NHPAI], 2000). Those practicing therapeutic touch are also encouraged to follow a code of ethics and conduct: practice must be consistent with the process Krieger and Kunz (1979) developed, obtain consent, respect the person's rights and responsibilities, and practice according to people's unique needs and individual differences (NHPAI, 2000).

A therapeutic touch session involves the clothed client sitting or lying down while the therapist passes his or her hands through the client's energy field, about two to three inches above the body. The therapist may or may not actually touch the client, but touch is not necessary. Sessions last no more than 30 minutes and consist of using touch to heal and relax the client (*Physician Desk Reference Health* [*PDR Health*], 2004).

Therapeutic touch practitioners undergo four phases in the process of therapeutic touch: centering, assessment, balancing, and reassessment (Brewer, 2004). Centering is focused on bringing your mind into a state of peace. Once the client is centered, the practitioner begins the second phase, assessment, by scanning the client's energy field to assess it for cues, which are the signs that guide the therapist. The practitioner does not make contact with the client when assessing the energy field because such touch may interfere with his or her ability to be aware of subtle cues. These cues are the essential pieces in the art of therapeutic touch. As the practitioner's ability to stay centered longer increases, intuitive cues in the form of hunches become more regular (Begley, 2001).

The third phase of balancing is done through a combination of several techniques that bring balance and harmony into the client's energy field. A few of the techniques used are modulating, tempering the energy outflow to the client needs, unruffling or clearing of the energy field to allow it to flow more smoothly, rebalancing of the field through opposite projections of given cues, and directing or transference of energy between different parts of the client's body. Relaxation is also gained through the use of a variety of mediums such as color, sound, visualization, or guided imagery. Reassessing, the final phase, determines whether the session has brought about the desired results. The preceding phases are not always used linearly, but are used in circular motion to produce the desired results (Begley, 2001).

The following case example is provided by Shirley Spear Begley, therapeutic touch practitioner and instructor.

Ana is a 63-year-old woman from Puerto Rico who had a total left knee replacement six months ago in the United States. She lives with her sister, who is present at the session and was the person who sought a therapist for therapeutic touch. Ana states she continues to be in considerable pain (rated 8 out of 10 when walking, and 4 out of 10 when resting). She has tried acupuncture, chiropractic, and a medical pain management clinic without pain relief. She was originally on narcotic analgesia, which she stopped because the medication made her sleepy and depressed. Occasionally she takes Darvocet for severe pain, yet is unable to take any anti-inflammatories due to a side effect of stomach upset. She is a former runner and in addition to the limitations in mobility, had to stop physical therapy rehabilitation for the knee, as it significantly exacerbated mid and low back pain. She has a history of mild scoliosis. Client tearfully states she has significant difficulty walking. She expressed frustration with her limitations and chronic pain and stated she is depressed. She appears retiring by nature and hesitant to share feelings, even with gentle prompting.

On therapeutic touch assessment, cues were perceived in upper back, central spine, and lumbar area as well as solar plexus, left groin, and inner aspect of left thigh and left knee. Client reported she felt a strong pain and heard a popping sound in left groin area some years ago when running a race and stopped running after that. The areas does not currently cause pain. Her left knee area is very warm to the touch both laterally and proximally. She states it has been that way since surgery. She does not have an energetic pulse in the left foot. All other areas are negative for cues.

TT, guided imagery, and breathwork was provided and methods for relaxation were taught. Ana did not express immediate relief, yet returned for five sessions, each time expressing greater relief and ease in walking that lasted after each session. Cues dissipated at end of each session, except heat in left knee that continued to be persistent, yet intermittent. By the third session, the client had returned to swimming and doing mild water aerobic activities. By the fifth session (over 26 days), she reported she was feeling very well and would be returning to Puerto Rico to care for her sister who was ill. She stated the sessions had provided "enormous relief and healing" and her sister concurred. At end of last session, when leaving, client expressed her gratitude for pain relief, emotional support and encouragement, smiled brightly, and spontaneously hugged therapist.

(S. Spear Begley, personal communication, June 2005)

Therapeutic touch is a recent therapy in the Western world, therefore research is scarce. Empirical research that exists regarding the clinical application of Reiki and therapeutic touch is found primarily in journals of nursing (Peters, 1999). Heidt (1981) conducted a study on the efficacy of therapeutic touch in a pre-post test quasi-experimental design. A sample of 90 hospitalized patients in a cardiovascular unit were separated into three groups: one that received therapeutic touch, one that received casual touch, and one that received no touch at all. The group receiving the therapeutic touch were given the four phases of touch therapy, the casual touch group had their vital signs checked by a therapist for an extended amount of time, and the no-touch group was simply asked questions about their feelings. Findings showed that patients in the therapeutic touch group demonstrated a significant decrease in anxiety level. In addition, results showed that patients in the therapeutic touch group exhibited a significantly greater decline in anxiety as compared to the casual and no-touch groups.

A study by Keller and Bzdek (1986) examined the effect of therapeutic touch in relation to intense tension headache pain. The sample consisted of 60 participants who were randomly assigned to either an experimental group that received therapeutic touch or a control group that received a placebo. In the placebo group, a nurse researcher mimicked the motions of therapeutic touch on a superficial level. Findings showed that 90 percent of subjects exposed to therapeutic touch experienced a significant reduction in headache immediately following the intervention and 70 percent maintained that decreased pain sensation four hours afterward. This pain reduction was significantly higher for the therapeutic touch group than the placebo group at both post testing and follow-up testing.

There are reports finding no benefits from therapeutic touch, however. Rose et al. (1998) tested the ability of therapeutic touch practitioners to correctly identify human fields. Under blinded conditions, practitioners were asked to identify which of their hands was closest to the investigator's hand. In only 44 percent of trials were the practitioners correct. Rosa et al. (1998) concluded that therefore "the claims of Therapeutic Touch are groundless and that further professional use is unjustified" (p. 1009).

Therefore, it appears that although many practitioners and clients believe that this complementary therapy is beneficial, the scientific community remains mixed at best in its support of therapeutic touch. This same controversy exists for most of the modalities considered complementary. Publications oriented to alternative practitioners such as massage therapists report a favorable view of the touch therapies, but these journals often publish less scientifically based research. It is important to encourage research regarding therapeutic touch as well as all of the complementary therapies.

MASSAGE AS TOUCH THERAPY

Unlike Reiki and therapeutic touch, massage is a manual manipulation that involves physically touching the body. According to the American Massage Therapy Association (AMTA), massage is described as a technique by which a practitioner uses his or her hands or body to manipulate soft tissue through holding, causing movement, or applying pressure to the body (AMTA, 2005). It is believed massage therapy can initiate certain physiological responses that reduce symptoms such as pain, stress, anxiety, and depression (Moyer, Rounds, & Hannum, 2004). The term "massage therapy" is considered an inclusive term for many therapies such as traditional therapeutic massage, acupressure, shiatsu, Thai, and ayurvedic massage as well as many more that go beyond the scope of this chapter.

In recent years the massage industry has grown in excess of $4 billion and has trained over 250,000 therapists. Twenty-seven percent of the adult population report having had treatment by a massage therapist in the past five years (AMTA, 2002). These numbers alone are a testament to the growing demand for massage as an effective touch therapy practice.

Massage has come full circle from its ancient beginnings and has been rediscovered in modern Western culture. Massage was introduced to the West through the creation of Swedish massage by Per Henrik Ling, the father of massage therapy (Calvert, 2002). Massage historians, such as Robert Calvert, author of *The History of Massage,* are cautious to bestow that honor to Ling because massage can be dated as early as 3000 BC. The Chinese have the oldest book written about massage, India practiced ayurvedic massage 4,000 years ago, the Egyptians speak clearly of reflexology, and Julius Caesar was believed to have received massage daily for neurological problems (Calvert, 2002). Massage eventually made a shift away from the medical establishment and went underground to become a popular folklore treatment. Henrik Ling and Dutch physician Metzger reversed this misfortune, and should receive proper credit for reintroducing massage to the medical society. It was from their work that other sub-specialties or systems of massage reemerged in the West.

Swedish massage, taught by Ling, is thought to be the most well-known and most widely practiced form of massage therapy. Most people receiving massage experience some application of Swedish technique. It is distinguished by its four touch techniques: stroking, kneading, striking, and rubbing (Calvert, 2002). Swedish massage can increase circulation to cleanse the body of toxins, release muscle tension, and improve the function of the organs and nervous system through the stroking of the skin. Swedish massage was one of the first techniques used to teach massage students and has since been the standard in massage schools. Today, Swedish massage is considered basic massage but according to Joe Lubow, director of the Sarasota School of Massage Therapy,

> Swedish massage is often not given enough credit for its therapeutic value. It was originally a rehabilitative treatment, but because massage schools incorporate it in their curriculum as a way of teaching the basic principle of massage, it has been unfairly reduced to a form of entry-level relaxation massage. It is not just a spring board for other systems, but a system of its own. (J. Lubow, personal communication, June 2005)

The National Institute of Health (NIH) has funded a clinical trial investigating the use of Swedish massage in treating fatigue in cancer patients undergoing chemotherapy (NIH, 2005) and while results are not yet reported, their interest encourages the use of massage therapy.

One of the most inclusive and cross cultural forms of massage is acupressure. Acupressure is based on the principle that the body has a system of energy channels, managed through pressure points, which, when blocked, can compromise normal body functions leading to illness or disease. Treatment involves applying pressure to specific points that are responsible for the flow of energy to a specific body part. Practitioners understand the body has a "map" of pressure points, each one related to a vital organ. Multiple points can be stimulated to ensure an optimal flow of energy throughout the whole body resulting in a renewed immune system and a feeling of well-being (Gach, 2004).

The theory of acupressure is a common thread through most Eastern healing systems. The Chinese refer to the pressure points as meridians and often refer to acupressure as needle-less acupuncture. In Japan, Shiatsu, meaning "finger pressure" uses hands, elbows, and feet to unlock the energy paths incorporated through a series of stretching techniques (Shiatsu Practitioners Association of Canada, 2005). Similarly, Thai massage integrates passive stretching, yoga postures, and pressure along energy lines to stimulate blocked energy and allow the body to recreate new energetic patterns and proper alignment. Finally, India's system of health, ayurveda, refers to the body's pressure points as "*marma* points" and applies acupressure, oil massage, aromatherapy, and energy healing to each point, opening the channels and restoring the body's normal functions. Despite its reputation as a noninvasive therapy, acupressure is reportedly powerful enough to rewire the body's central nervous system. In Pan Nain's documentary *Ayurveda: The Art of Being,* a doctor demonstrated the power behind the technique by paralyzing a goat after touching a *marma* point on the back of his skull. Specialists in acupressure would argue that the healing power of all massage techniques come from some form of stimulation to pressure points.

In recent years, the field of massage therapy has benefited from research activities intended to understand how massage affects the body. Organizations such as the Touch Research Institute (TRI), part of the University of Miami School of Medicine, have been pioneers in expanding the use of massage and supporting the treatment with research. TRI has conducted over 90 research projects investigating the use of massage in illnesses ranging from Alzheimer's to substance abuse. This institute found positive results using massage for infant weight gain, immune functioning for patients with diseases such as HIV and cancer, and pain reduction in fibromyalgia (Field, 2000). According to TRI, most of the healing occurs from the decrease in stress hormones.

In addition, the National Institute of Health (NIH) is conducting clinical trials to determine the benefits of massage for treatment in depression, cancer-related fatigue, and immune system functioning. NIH has funded a study of massage as an intervention for pain relief and depression during end of life, coordinating the efforts of 12 hospice facilities across the country to investigate the therapeutic use of massage (NIH, 2005). NIH has established the National Center for Complementary and Alternative Medicine (NCCAM) which is actively involved in funding and publishing research activities in massage therapy.

ETHICAL AND LEGAL ISSUES

To ensure confidence and safety in the therapeutic practice, professional organizations and state licensing boards establish ethical and regulatory guidelines for the appropriate use of touch. Because the use of touch in therapy is a sensitive issue that carries potential risk, ethical and legal guidelines are essential to maintaining the integrity of the therapy and protection of the client.

The National Association for Social Workers (NASW) and the American Psychological Association (APA) have both developed ethical guidelines to ensure that practitioners meet professional standards and each have clear positions on the role and limits of touch. The NASW (1996) in its recent revision of the *Code of Ethics* included a stronger worded guideline than in past editions:

> Social workers should not engage in physical contact with clients when there is a possibility of psychological harm to the client as a result of the contact (such as cradling or caressing clients). Social workers who engage in appropriate physical contact with clients are responsible for setting clear, appropriate, and culturally sensitive boundaries that govern such physical contact. (Section 1.10, p. 13)

Some social workers often require clients to sign an Informed Consent to establish the intent and permission to touch. The consent form will typically identify the treatment, its objectives, and any potential harmful effects. The APA is involved in establishing ethics, licensure, and accreditation, a unique combination that provides a powerful voice to their ethical expectations. While the APA does not address the use of touch as therapeutic, section 10 of the *Ethical Principles of Psychologist and Code of Conduct* creates a definitive line between an appropriate use of touch and unethical sexual relationships (APA, 2002). These ethical standards benefit both the therapist and the client by providing professional guidelines for the therapist and protecting the client from inappropriate and harmful behavior.

Similar to psychotherapy, massage therapy, Reiki, and therapeutic touch publish a code of ethics intended to protect the well-being of the client. Each of these therapies has a professional association that has voluntarily established ethical guidelines and boundaries necessary to touch a client. While most incorporate the guidelines for touch under the category of professional behavior and respect for the individual, the International Association of Reiki Professionals provides very specific ethical guidelines for restricting touch from parts of the body that may be erotic or sexually charged. Although none of these associations play a legal role nor require membership to practice, they do act as a professional watchtower and can be either a referral base for qualified professionals or an avenue for reporting inappropriate or unprofessional behavior.

State and local agencies are responsible for establishing the licensing regulations for practice and providing recourse when harm is suspected. Advocates for CAM have expressed concern over stringent licensing requirements that may restrict access to CAM therapies and state authorities work to maintain this balance. This chapter presents licensing requirements for massage, Reiki, and therapeutic touch (see Table 10.1). Thirty-three states and the District of Columbia require massage therapists to be licensed by the state and meet specific standards for education and testing (AMTA, 2005). While there is no license for therapeutic touch, most practitioners are licensed health care professionals. The Nurse Healers-Professional Associates (NHPA), a professional association for therapeutic touch, strongly recommends that individuals without a health care license limit their therapy practice to family, friends, and religious groups (NHPA, 2005). Reiki, as a profession has no national licensure requirements, but in recent years has found itself in contentious debates with states and massage boards over the lack of licensure. As of 2001, three states—Florida, North Dakota, and Massachusetts require Reiki professionals to be licensed massage therapists while 20 states do not consider Reiki part of massage therapy and therefore have eliminated them from the massage licensing standards (Sacred Path, 2001). The remaining states are still considering the issue.

TABLE 10.1. Licensing Requirements for Massage, Reiki, and Therapeutic Touch

Profession	Professional Association Code of Ethics	State Licensing Requirements	Web Site Information
Psychology	American Psychological Association (APA)[a]	State license required to practice psychology.	www.apa.org
Social Work	National Association of Social Workers (NASW)[a]	State license required to practice social work. For a list of licensing boards by state go to www.swes.net/licensing/boards.html	www.naswdc.org
Therapeutic Touch	Nurse Healers-Professional Associates International	None—although, most are licensed health care professionals	www.therapeutic touch.org
Reiki	International Association of Reiki Professionals[a]	State by state guidelines. Contact a local health department	www.iarp.org
Massage Therapy	American Massage Therapy Association[a]	33 states and DC require state license to practice. For a state list go to www.amtamassage.org	www.amtamasage.org

[a]Association offers liability insurance.

Using touch with clients is varied and controversial, however the results are often beneficial. The intervention ranges from ancient times to present, from actual touch to aura touch, from Western medicine to Eastern chakra touch, and from psychological touch to physical touch. All forms of touch described here—touch in psychotherapy, Reiki, therapeutic touch, and massage therapy—are intended to increase the well-being of the client and enhance the mind-body connection.

REFERENCES

American Massage Therapy Association. (2002). Demand for massage therapy. Retrieved July 25, 2005, from www.amtamassage.org.
American Massage Therapy Association. (2005). Credentials for massage therapy professions. Retrieved July 25, 2005, from www.amtamassage.org.

American Massage Therapy Association. (2005). Definition of massage therapy. Retrieved July 25, 2005, from www.amtamassage.org.

American Psychological Association. (2002). Ethical principles of psychologists and code of conduct. Retrieved June 3, 2005, from www.apa.org.

Bacorn, C.N. & Dixon, D.N. (1984). The effects of touch on depressed and vocationally undecided clients. *Journal of Counseling Psychology, 31,* 488-496.

Begley, S.S. (January/February, 1999). Feeling the flow: The energetic language of therapeutic touch. *Massage Magazine,* 59-71.

Brewer, A.V. (2005, May 3). Complementary and alternative medicine: A physician's guide. Energy healing. Retrieved May 3, 2005, from http://medicine.wustl.edu/~compmed/cam_ene.html.

Calvert, R. (2002). *The History of Massage.* Vermont: Healing Arts Press.

Chan, P. (2005). Reiki and the conventional health care provider recommendations and potholes. The International Center for Reiki Training. Retrieved July 23, 2005, from www.reiki.org.

Cohen, S.S. (1986). *The magic of touch.* New York, NY: Harper & Row.

Durana, C. (1998). The use of touch in psychotherapy: Ethical and clinical guidelines. *Psychotherapy, 35*(2), 269-280.

Ferenczi, S. (1933). The confusion of tongues between adults and children: The language of tenderness and passion. In M. Balint (Ed.), *Final contributions to the problems and methods of psycho-analysis* (Vol. 3 ed., pp. 156-167). New York: Brunner/Mazel.

Field, T. (2000). *Touch therapy.* London: Churchill Livingstone.

Field, T., Schanberg, S., Scafidi, F., Bauer, C., Vega-Lehr, N., Garcia, R., Nystrom, J., & Kuhn, C. (1986). Tactile/kinesthetic stimulation effects on preterm neonates. *Pediatrics, 77,* 654-658.

Fuchs, L.L. (1975). Reflections on touching and transference in psychotherapy. *Clinical Social Work Journal, 3,* 167-176.

Gach, M.R. (2004). *Acupressure.* London, England: Piatkus Books.

Heidt, P. (1981). The effects of therapeutic touch on anxiety level of hospitalized patients. *Nursing Research, 30,* 32-37.

Hunter, M. & Struve, J. (1998). *The ethical use of touch in psychotherapy.* Three Oaks, CA: Sage Publications.

International Association of Reiki Professionals. (1997). Retrieved May 2, 2005, from www.iarp.org.

International Association of Reiki Professionals. (2003). Retrieved March 30, 2007, from www.iarp.org.

International Association of Reiki Professionals. (2005). Retrieved March 30, 2007, from www.iarp.org.

Jourard, S. & Friedman, R. (1970). Experimentor-subject distance and self-disclosure. *Journal of Personality and Social Psychology, 14*(3), 278-282.

Keller, E. & Bzdek, V.M. (1986). Effects of therapeutic touch on tension headache pain. *Nursing Research, 35*(2), 101-105.

Kertay, L. & Reviere, S.L. (1993). The use of touch in psychotherapy: Theoretical and ethical considerations. *Psychotherapy, 30*(1), 32-40.

Kiernan, J. (2002). The experience of therapeutic touch in the lives of five postpartum women. *The American Journal of Maternal Child Nursing, 27*(1), 47-53.

Krieger, D. & Kunz, D. (1979). *The therapeutic touch: How to use your hands to help or heal.* Engelwood Cliffs, NJ: Prentice Hall, Inc.

Kupfermann, K. & Smaldino, C. (1987). The vitalizing and revitalizing experience of reliability: The place of touch in psychotherapy. *Clinical Social Work Journal, 15*(3), 223-235.

Lipinski, K. (2005). Enhancing nursing practice with Reiki. The International Center for Reiki Training. Retrieved July 23, 2005, from www.reiki.org.

Macrae, J. (1987). *Theraputic touch: A practical guide.* New York: Alfred A. Knoff, Inc. & Random House, Inc.

Milakovich, J.C. (1998). Differences between therapists who touch and those who do not. In E.W.L. Smith, P.R. Clance, & S. Imes, *Touch in therapy. theory, research, and practice* (pp. 74-91). New York: Guilford.

Mintz, E.E. (1969). On the rationale of touch in psychotherapy. *Psychotherapy: Theory, Research, and Practice, 6*(4), 232-234.

Moyer, C., Rounds, J., & Hannum, J., (2004). A meta-analysis of massage therapy research. *Psychological Bulletin, 130*(1), 3-18.

National Association of Social Workers. (1996). *Code of ethics.* Washington, DC: NASW.

National Institute of Health. (2005). *Massage therapy for cancer related fatigue.* Retrieved March 30, 2007, from http://clinicaltrials.gov/show/NCT00039793.

Nurse Healers-Professional Associates International (NHPA). (1995). Statement of ethics and conduct for the practice of therapeutic touch. Retrieved June 2, 2005, from www.therapeutic-touch.org.

Nurse Healers-Professional Associates International (NHPA). (2000). Retrieved May 3, 2005, from www.therapeutic-touch.org.

Nurse Healers-Professional Associates International (NHPA). (2005). Retrieved March 30, 2007, from www.therapeutic-touch.org.

Older, J. (1977). Four taboos that may limit the success of psychotherapy. *Psychiatry, 40,* 197-204.

Older, J. (1982). *Touching is healing.* New York: Stein & Day.

Pattison, E.J. (1973). Effects of touch on self-exploration and the therapeutic relationship. *Journal of Consulting and Clinical Psychology, 40,* 170-175.

PDRhealth. 2004. Thomas Healthcare. Retrieved May 3, 2005, from www.pdrhealth .com/content/natural_medicine/chapters/201480.shtml.

Pederson, D. (1973). Self-disclosure, body accessibility, and personal space. *Psychological Reports, 33,* 975-980.

Peters, R.M. (1999). The effectiveness of therapeutic touch: A meta-analytic review. *Nursing Science Quarterly, 12*(1), 52-61.

Rand, W. (1991). *Reiki the healing touch: First and second degree manual.* Southfield, MI: Vision Publications.

Rosa, L., Rosa, E., Sarner, L., & Barrett, S. (1998). A close look at therapeutic touch. *The Journal of the American Medical Association, 279*(1), 1005-1010.

Sacred Path. (2001). The national status of reiki laws by state. Retrieved June 2, 2005, from www.sacredpath.org.

Shiatsupractitioner's Association of Canada. (2005). About shiatsu. Retrieved April 13, 2005, from www.shiatsupractor.org.

Smith, E., Clance, P., & Imes, S. (1998). *Touch in psychotherapy.* New York: Guilford Press.

Spear Beagley, S. (2005). Personal communication.

Spotnitz, H. (1972). Touch countertransference in group psychotherapy. *International Journal of Group Psychotherapy, 22,* 455-463.

Stein, D. (1990). *All women are healers: A comprehensive guide to natural healing.* Freedom, CA: The Crossing Press.

Strozier, A., Krizek, C., & Sale, K. (2000). [Touch study]. Unpublished raw data.

Strozier, A., Krizek, C., & Sale, K. (2003). Touch: Its use in psychotherapy. *Journal of Social Work Practice, 17*(1), 49-62.

Wilson, J.M. (1982). The value of touch in psychotherapy. *American Journal of Orthopsychiatry, 52*(1), 65-72.

Wilson, B.G. & Masson, R.L. (1986). The role of touch in therapy: An adjunct to communication. *Journal of Counseling and Development, 64,* 497-500.

Appendix

Resources for Further Exploration

The following are resources that you may find helpful in exploring one or more of these complementary and alternative therapies in more depth.

RESOURCES FOR MINDFULNESS (CHAPTER 2)

Professional Associations

The Mind and Life Institute: The Mind and Life Institute [MLI] was cofounded in 1987 by the Dalai Lama, neuroscientist Francisco J. Varela, and entrepreneur Adam Engle for the purpose of creating a rigorous dialogue and research collaboration between modern science, and Buddhism. The MLI operates through four divisions: meetings and dialogues, publications, scientific education, and research grants/sponsorship. Since 2000, the primary focus of the MLI has been the creation of a new interdisciplinary field of science that asks and answers the question: how do we create and maintain a healthy mind?

www.mindandlife.org

Media Source

Sounds True: Audio, Video, and Music for the Inner Life

Contact:
Boulder, Colorado 1-800-333-9185
www.soundstrue.com

Periodicals

What Is Enlightenment?

Moksha Press
Andrew Cohen, Editor-in-Chief
www.wie.org

Introduction to Alternative and Complementary Therapies
© 2008 by The Haworth Press, Taylor & Francis Group. All rights reserved.
doi:10.1300/5987_11

271

Shambhala Sun—Buddhism Culture Meditation Life

Contact:
Melvin McLeod, Editor-in-Chief
1345 Spruce Street
Boulder, CO 80302-4886
www.shambhalasun.com

Tricycle, the Buddhist Review

Contact:
The Buddhist Ray, Inc.
P.O. Box 2077
Marion, OH 43306
www.tricycle.com

Spirituality and Health—The Soul/Body Connection

Contact:
Peter D. Wild, Publisher
P.O. Box 54151
Boulder, CO 80322-4151
www.SpiritualityHealth.com

The Institute of Noetic Sciences: This site explores the frontiers of consciousness to advance individual, social, and global transformation.

Contact:
Petaluma, CA 707-775-3500
www.noetic.org

Internet Resources

Duke Center for Integrative Medicine: This site provides information about the Mindfulness-Based Stress Reduction Program.

www.dcim.org

Center for Mindfulness, UMass Medical School: This group originated and is the national model for Mindfulness-Based Stress Reduction programs.

www.umassmed.edu/cfm

Mind and Life Institute: This group is well known for its meetings and conferences involving leading Western scientists and healers, H.H. the Dalai Lama, and others interested in contemplative approaches to modern life.

www.mindandlife.org

Dharma: This site contains information about *Vipassana* retreat centers and schedules. *Vipassana* is a name for the practice of mindfulness meditation in the *Theravada* branch of Buddhism. The meditation instructions are very simple, and have been the basis for a number of the mindfulness programs that are currently offered in Western clinical settings.

www.dharma.org

RESOURCES FOR SPIRITUALITY (CHAPTER 3)

Professional Associations

The Society for Spirituality and Social Work: This society addresses issues related to a wide variety of religious and nonreligious forms of spirituality through networking, conferences, and publications.

http://ssw.asu.edu/spirituality/ssw

Canadian Association for Spirituality and Social Work: This association holds national conferences addressing spirituality and social work in Canada.

http://www/cnssw.org

North American Society for Christians and Social Work: This organization addresses spirituality from a Christian perspective through conferences and publications.

Contact:
P.O. Box 121 Botsford, CT 0604-0121
www.nascw.org

National Association for Jewish Communal Professionals: This is an organization for social workers employed by a variety of Jewish social service organizations.

Study Center

Center for Spirituality and Integral Social Work (CSISW): This center was developed by the National Catholic School of Social Service. The CSISW is dedicated to providing integrated state-of-the-art social work research, training, and service from a bio-psycho-social-spiritual perspective, with a particular emphasis on spirituality, guided by integral theory.

http://csisw.cua.edu

Journals

Journal of Religion and Spirituality in Social Work (formerly *Social Thought*)

Published by The Haworth Press.
This journal publishes a variety of articles addressing religion, spirituality, and ethics.

Social Work and Christianity: An International Journal

This journal is published by the North American Association of Christians in Social Work and contains articles related to spirituality, religion, and social work.

RESOURCES FOR POETRY (CHAPTER 4)

Professional Association

National Association for Poetry Therapy: The purpose of this organization is to support the field of poetry therapy through specific projects, and it has created both long- and short-term programs to support research, education, projects, training, and clinical practice in poetry therapy.

www.poetrytherapy.org

Internet Resources

The Poetry Practice: This site emphasizes writing in your own way and assists the user to write in his or her voice in a manner that promotes hope and healing.

www.poetrypractice.com

Poetic Medicine: This site encourages the browser to use a wide range of creative tools and techniques that can act as a healing catalyst such as the reading and writing of poems.

www.poeticmedicine.com

RESOURCES FOR ART THERAPY (CHAPTER 5)

Professional Association

American Art Therapy Association: This organization is composed of professionals dedicated to the belief that the creative process involved in the making of art is healing and life-enhancing. Its mission is to serve its members and the general public by providing standards of professional competence, and developing and promoting knowledge in, and of, the field of art therapy.

www.arttherapy.org

Internet Resources

Arts and Healing Network: This site is an online resource for anyone interested in the healing potential of art.

www.artheals.org

Art Therapy Credentials Board (ATCB): This is an independent organization that, after reviewing documentation of completion of graduate education and postgraduate supervised experience, grants postgraduate registration (ATR). The Registered Art Therapist who successfully completes the written examination administered by the ATCB is qualified as Board Certified (ATR-BC).

www.atcb.org

RESOURCES FOR PSYCHODRAMA (CHAPTER 6)

Professional Associations

The American Board of Examiners: This association has established national professional standards in the field of psychodrama, sociometry, and group psychotherapy. The Board has established two levels of certification: the first is the Practitioner (CP) level and the subsequent is the Trainer, Educator, and Practitioner (TEP) level. Certification in either level requires considerable supervised experience, an examination, and an onsite observation. The Board of Examiners annually publishes the *Directory and Certification Standards* that describes detailed training requirements and lists certified practitioners and trainers by region.

Contact:
Dale Richard Buchanan, PhD
The American Board of Examiners in Psychodrama,
Sociometry and Group Psychotherapy
P.O. Box 15572
Washington, DC 20003-0572
Phone: (201) 483-0514

The American Society for Group Psychotherapy and Psychodrama (ASGPP): This organization is an interdisciplinary membership organization that supports the development of psychodrama in clinical and community practice, teaching, research, and training. The ASGPP sets ethical standards, holds national and regional conferences, and publishes the *Journal of Group Psychotherapy, Psychodrama, and Sociometry.*

Contact:
301 N. Harrison Street, Suite 508
Princeton, NJ 08540
Phone: (609) 452-1339
Fax: (609) 936-1659
E-mail: asgpp@asgpp.org
Website: www.asgpp.org

International Association of Group Psychotherapy (IAGP): This organization is a worldwide network of professionals involved in the development of group psychotherapy in the areas of theory, clinical practice, training, research, and consultancy.

www.iagp.com

Journal

The Journal of Group Psychotherapy, Psychodrama, and Sociometry **(formerly *The International Journal of Action Methods*)**

Heldref publications www.heldref.org

RESOURCES FOR DANCE MOVEMENT THERAPY (CHAPTER 7)

Professional Association

American Dance Therapy Association: This national association disseminates information about the DMT field. It also provides a list of graduate programs leading to the MA in DMT which have earned the association's "Approval" status. Information about alternate route training may also be obtained from this association.

Contact:
American Dance Therapy Association
2000 Century Plaza, Suite 108
10632 Little Patuxent Parkway
Columbia, MD 21044-3263
Phone: (410) 997-4040
E-mail: info@adta.org

Journals

American Journal of Dance Therapy: This is a national professional journal that publishes professional articles in the DMT field.

Published by Human Sciences Press, New York

Arts in Psychotherapy Journal: This is an international and interdisciplinary journal that publishes professional articles from the creative arts therapy field which encompasses art therapy, dance therapy, drama therapy, music therapy, and poetry therapy.

Published by Elsevier Science, New York

RESOURCES FOR MUSIC THERAPY (CHAPTER 8)

Professional Associations

American Music Therapy Association: This organization is dedicated to the advancement of public awareness of the benefits of music therapy and is the governing body for music therapists in the United States.

www.musictherapy.org

Association for Music and Imagery: This organization is comprised of persons trained in The Bonny Method of Guided Imagery and Music.

www.bonnymethod.com/ami/index.html

Internet Resources

Bonny Institute: This institute provides the history and development of the Bonny Method of Guided Imagery and Music.

www.bonnyinstitute.org

Certification Board for Music Therapists: This board is an independent body that credentials music therapists who have completed academic and clinical training and also tracks continuing education of credentialed professionals.

www.cbmt.org

World Federation of Music Therapy: This federation is the only international organization dedicated to the development of music therapy worldwide.

http://musictherapyworld.net

Voices: This site is a world forum for music therapy and includes columns, essays, and discussions.

www.voices.no

RESOURCES FOR ANIMAL-ASSISTED THERAPY (CHAPTER 9)

Professional Associations

The Delta Society: This society has been instrumental in advancing the standard definitions in the field today, distinguishing between animal-assisted activities (AAA) and animal-assisted therapy (AAT).

www.deltasociety.org

Center to Study Human Animal Relationships and Environments (CENSHARE): CENSHARE is a diverse group of people from the University of Minnesota and the surrounding community dedicated to studying and improving human-animal relationships and environments. CENSHARE'S mission includes education, research, and service.

www.censhare.umn.edu

Internet Resource

Animal-Assisted Therapy and Animal-Assisted Activities (AAT/AAA): This site explores the world of animal-assisted therapy and animal-assisted activities.

www.animaltherapy.net

RESOURCES FOR TOUCH THERAPY (CHAPTER 10)

Professional Associations

The Official Organization of Therapeutic Touch: The mission of this organization is to lead, inspire, and advance excellence in Krieger and Kunz Therapeutic Touch as a healing practice and lifeway.

www.therapeutic-touch.org

Healing Touch International, Inc.: The purpose of the Healing Touch International Foundation is to receive and distribute funds to assist, encourage, and advance the philosophy, objectives and techniques of healing touch therapy and other energy-based healing therapies.

www.healingtouch.net

Internet Resource

Therapeutic Touch: This site defines therapeutic touch, gives the history of the therapy, provides information on being both a patient and therapist of touch therapy, and gives information on upcoming workshops.

www.therapeutictouch.org

Videos

Therapeutic Touch: The Vision & The Reality (19 minutes, NH-PAI, 1995).

The Role of the Physical, Mental & Spiritual Bodies in Healing, Dora Kunz (47 minutes, NH-PAI, 1997).

Index

Page numbers followed by the letter "t" indicate tables.